Redeeming Childbirth

Experiencing His Presence in Pregnancy, Labor, Childbirth, and Beyond

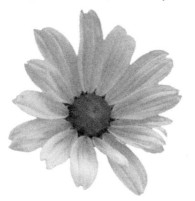

Angie Tolpin

AngieTolpin.com
RedeemingChildbirth.com

This book provides information and stories about alternative approaches to pregnancy and childbirth care.
It's contents were current to the best of the author's knowledge at the time of its publication. Before following
any advice contained within its contents, the reader should verify the information and make decisions with
the guidance of their own health care provider, physician, or midwife. The information provided in this
book is based upon in-depth research of current medical literature and interviews with acknowledged
experts in the field. This book is intended only as a resource for spiritual encouragement. The author and
publisher are not responsible for any adverse effects resulting from the use of the information contained in
this book.

ISBN-10: 0-9852463-1-6
ISBN-13: 978-0-9852463-1-0

Library of Congress Control Number: 2012923317

Printed in the United States of America

Some photos, including the cover photo by A Little Rojo alittlerojo.com.
Cover design idea by Erin Ulrich @ Design by Insight designbyinsight.net.
Edited by Sandra Peoples @ Next Step Editing nextstepediting.com

Dedication

I dedicate this book to my Deliverer and Savior Jesus Christ, and to all my children. It is because of what Jesus has done in my life through your births that I am able to share *Redeeming Childbirth*.

Leaving a legacy is my deepest passion as a mother and woman of God. I pray that when I am no longer on this earth, this message the Lord has blessed my heart with will encourage and equip sisters in the faith for generations to come. As a woman who desires to bring truth and strength to the next generation of mothers, my passion and prayer is that I can empower them to be strong women in the Lord and to embrace the unique design God has made in them.

Give Him your best in all you do, for His glory.

> For the Lord God has said,
> *"Behold, children are a heritage from the Lord,
> the fruit of the womb a reward." Psalm 127:3*

May your labors of love draw you closer to your Savior, husband, children, and other women in your life. The bond between mother and child is so precious, may we embrace each moment with them from the very start of their lives.

May you experience His presence and grow in faith, hope, and love.

Endorsements

Angie presents a biblical perspective on pain and trials—they are a blessing and a means of grace. I have not come across another book that so clearly reveals God's work in the family through the gift of childbirth.

-Vergil Brown,
Lead Pastor at Gresham Bible Church

Angie casts a beautiful vision for making Christ the center of your pregnancy and childbirth. She brings a unique perspective on the redeeming power of pain to challenge her readers to rethink their own ideas. Angie calls out the disunity amongst Christian sisters over birth methods. Through her own birth stories and those of others, Angie shows how God can be glorified in hospital rooms and birthing centers alike. A refreshing read for moms old and new! Even if you're not expecting, it will challenge your relationship with your Savior and with your family.

-Gretchen Louise,
farmer's wife and mother of three,
editor at the Young Ladies Christian Fellowship

I was so blessed to be able to read Redeeming Childbirth before my birth. Although I am a Christian and I had confidence in my ability to birth my baby, I hadn't been preparing to experience God and HIS presence in my birth. Angie's encouragement to make a conscience decision to have God be a part of every aspect of the pregnancy and birth changed my perspective. I was inspired to print Bible verses and phrases I planned to read during labor and was looking forward to experiencing God in a new way. I would recommend this book to every mama-to-be.

-Robin Dufel,
first time mama

I wish we had this book years ago. Angie's approach to pregnancy, childbirth, and the sovereignty of God would have really saved my wife and me from much pain when we had our miscarriages. Men should absolutely read this book, not just moms, and I can't wait to share Angie's message with our kids when the time is right.

-Trent Booth, Pastor,
LifeWalk Church

Contents

Part IV

Part V

Foreword

Expecting a baby is such an exciting season. It's a time to dream about your little one, a time to prepare your heart for the upcoming joys and challenges of parenting, and a time to depend on God.

I absolutely love babies and I love being a mom. I just love pulling-off darling baby-booties and kissing those tiny toes. I wonder where those feet may go and I think about God's future plans. It's remarkable how such a little person can make such a big impact.

A few days ago I attended a baby shower and as I prepared my gift, I thought about *Redeeming Childbirth*, and how I long for the day when I can buy a stack of this book. What a blessing for a new expectant mother, to provide her what she really needs: encouragement from a sweet friend, spiritual wisdom, and guidance to trust in God.

Angie Tolpin has done a wonderful job in writing *Redeeming Childbirth, Experiencing His Presence in Pregnancy, Labor, Birth, and Beyond*. This book is a much-needed blessing, for families and for churches. It's a book to encourage pregnant mothers to grow in their relationships with the Lord, and to encourage unity among Christian women in regard to the many issues of childbirth.

As a mother of six, Angie is definitely qualified to write this book. But even more importantly, I believe she has been called to write it. For years, Angie has felt compelled to seek God and to gather spiritual encouragement and hope for expectant mothers (and their husbands). Throughout all of her pregnancies, Angie journaled her thoughts and her prayers, with a vision to someday write this book and to mentor new mothers. Her desire to help you during your pregnancy has been a growing burden and a vision. In the midst of her busy life—supporting her husband, speaking at marriage seminars, raising and home schooling her children, and living for Jesus—Angie has been thinking about you. She has prayed for you and has poured-out her heart on these pages. Consider that thought for a moment. For years, God has been thinking about YOU and your upcoming birth. YOU have been on God's heart. He loves you and wants you to experience His presence and His joy. As your baby grows inside you, God wants your relationship with Him to grow too!

During pregnancy, all of the unknowns and details can seem overwhelming; but God desires to be with you and to help you. Even if you don't yet know Him in a personal way, be assured God knows you and He loves you very much. Jesus cares about you and your baby, and He wants to become your closest friend.

In the Bible, we are encouraged to follow the example of Jesus Christ. Hebrews 12:1-2 says, ". . . let us run with endurance the race that is set before us, looking unto Jesus, the author and finisher of our faith, who for the joy that was set before Him endured the cross . . ." As a pregnant mother, the nine-month challenge of pregnancy, ending with labor and delivery, can feel like a challenge and perhaps like a cross to bear. But consider how Jesus endured His cross . . . with JOY. Jesus focused on the purpose of the cross—paying the penalty for the sins of the world and providing His salvation. As mothers, we too can take up our crosses . . . with JOY! With God's help, we can focus on the purpose of our pregnancies. What a joy to carry precious children in our wombs and to deliver babies into this world. What a joy to love and to nurture little ones. And what an awesome responsibility to teach and to train a child, day-by-day, in the way he or she should go.

May God bless your birth and all that is ahead.

Ann Dunagan

Author of *The Mission Minded Family, The Mission Minded Child, and Scarlet Cord: Nothing but the Blood of Jesus*

Ann is a homeschooling mother of seven, an international speaker with *HarvestMinistry.org*, co-founder of an orphanage ministry (caring for over 700 children), and founder of *DaringDaughters.org*.

Second Foreword

The birth of a child is so much more than a physiological response and sequence that began when two loving people shared an intimate moment and ended in the bright lights of a delivery suite in a hospital. It is a process that has great spiritual significance for everyone involved.

As the mother of six children, and as a woman who birthed her children in different settings and different circumstances, we can trust Angie's guidance and experience. Her experience was not only the catalyst for this book but also the driving passion to see all women be restored to a strong faith in how God marvelously designed their bodies. Aside from her own experiences, Angie also engaged other mothers, gathered the wisdom of many women and childbirth experts, and has presented us with bushels and baskets overflowing with wisdom and stories of positive life-affirming experiences in hospital birth rooms, birth centers, and home births.

The awareness that the mother and baby dyad are doing a sacred job is often missing in the birth room. We focus so much on the physical that we forget the spiritual. We leave God at home. We trust God in our lives, to the best of our ability, to govern our decisions about money, career, marriage, even finding a house and where we live. But, most couples forget that in this one area it is the MOST important time to remember God's presence and invite Him into the labor and birth process. Angie and Isaac did that, praying openly and asking God to be with them during the birth. I am always thrilled when I am able to serve couples who embrace God and welcome His presence in the birth room. It was an honor and privilege to witness Angie's strength and the way she surrendered as her labor progressed and her daughter was born.

Hours before the baby was born, as I arrived at the hospital, I sat in the parking lot in my car and asked for God's divine guidance during this birth. I often will pray before a birth, "These are your eyes, Lord; let me use them to see only the good in every situation and to notice the subtle ways this mother and father and baby will be communicating nonverbally. These are your lips, Lord; let me speak only when necessary and with words of truth and beauty. These are your feet, Lord; let them take me to the right place at the right time. These are your hands, Lord; let me use them in ways to bring comfort."

As health care professionals we should ask, "How can we best support the mother to 'let the baby' out, honor the natural processes, and enhance the connection between mother and baby, before, during and after the birth?" This question is faithfully answered through the tips, testimonies, prayers, and Scriptures Angie shares. The hope and faith in God this book will encourage you to have will inspire you to think different about birth.

Thank you, Angie, for so eloquently reminding us through *Redeeming Childbirth* to reconnect and recommit to the sacredness of birth and motherhood. "Wisdom will enter your heart, and knowledge will fill you with joy. Wise choices will watch over you. Understanding will keep you safe" (Proverbs 2:10-11, NLT).

Barbara Harper October 20, 2012

Author of *Gentle Birth Choices*
RN, CLD, CCCE, Founder of Waterbirth International, Angie's first midwife!
waterbirth.org

Letter from Author

Throughout the Old Testament, our forefathers built altars for the Lord God. They often built these altars after they had experienced God in a merciful and compassionate way.

In Genesis 12:7, "Then the LORD appeared to Abram and said, 'To your offspring I will give this land.' So he built there an altar to the LORD, who had appeared to him." Abram built the altar because the Lord had appeared to him and blessed him.

Because Jesus died on the cross and paid the final penalty for all our sins, as Christians we no longer have a need to sacrifice or burn offerings at an altar. Jesus was that sacrifice, that offering; He paid for it all. Since we no longer need to build an altar for sacrifice, when the Lord blesses us or has been merciful, we rob ourselves of a spiritual blessing. Those altars represented God's provision and mercy. Without them we are quick to forget His goodness. This year I was humbled to acknowledge that the amount of thanksgiving I pour out in honor of what God has done in my life is far smaller than building an altar. In the Scriptures, after an altar was built, the men of old experienced an intimate time with the Lord, communicating with Him, worshiping Him, and meditating in awe of God's majesty.

We are set free in Christ and in relationship with Him, so we can experience an intimate conversation with Him from anywhere, anytime, without the need to build an altar. However, we can potentially miss out on the blessing of intimacy with Christ that comes from physically dedicating ourselves to a service like building an altar. The kind of service that flows from a heart filled with gratitude for what He alone has done.

An altar served as a reminder of what God had done. Years after having built an altar, these prophets of old would be reminded of the great works and love of the Lord when they came upon these holy places. Often times, they built alters after being delivered and saved from the hands of an enemy or saved from events such as the great flood. Many altars were built to remind them of God's acts of deliverance.

The Lord has shown Himself a great deliverer in my births as He provided physical strength to endure and persevere. The Lord took something that could have been simply a means to an end (pain in return for the blessing of a child) and He redeemed my experiences, making them meaningful milestones in my spiritual journey. *Redeeming Childbirth* is my way of thanking the Lord for how He has blessed me. It is my altar to remember the great things He continues to do in the lives of those who love Him, for it shall remind me of the works of the Lord in my life and for His saving grace, both in birth and eternal life.

When I was a young girl, my pastor, Pastor Roluffs, used to say, "We are blessed to be a blessing." That has stuck with me my whole life. Blessed to be a blessing. The Lord blessed me in my births, now it's my turn to bless others and bless His holy name. God cares for us so much that He wants us to benefit from having a deeper understanding of His goodness by experiencing His grace and who He is. But He also allows us to learn lessons for the benefit of others as well. We are blessed to be a blessing. His blessings are not necessarily just for us, but to be shared.

Out of a deep desire and passion to fulfill an act of obedience to my Father in heaven, I am stepping out in this journey to write for Him. For years I have felt a yearning to share with you my personal experience of connecting with God in childbirth. Shortly after I gave birth to my first daughter in 2000, I immediately felt His call to share the gift of understanding with others.

After every subsequent birth I felt empowered by God to write, but the reality of my humanity humbled me, creating doubt that anyone would listen. So I journaled, studied the Word, prayed and waited, knowing I had so much more to learn from the Lord. Years passed, I had more babies, and every time I felt the Lord tugging at me to stand up and share a message of empowerment and hope. A message that I frequently needed to remind myself of, but felt it was not yet His timing. During all those years it was my feelings of inadequacy that prevented me from taking action. I would get discouraged and listen to those whispers of doubt in my mind saying women didn't need this message.

I thought, "Who am I Lord?" It finally occurred to me that while humility is good, inaction is not. Especially when that action is a calling by God. The Lord has made it abundantly clear to me that even though I still feel inadequate and am equally aware of my own need for growth, He has called me to this act of obedience at this specific time.

In an attempt to purposefully mentor women toward seeking God and inviting Him into their birthing experiences, I am excited to journey through the Scriptures with you on topics such as:

- What redeeming childbirth means and what it looks like.
- Lies women believe and false teachings about birth.
- Fears that bind us.
- Preparing your heart, soul, and mind for birth and motherhood.
- Experiencing the presence of the Lord in birth through prayer and worship.
- Being a missionary wherever you are, even in the midst of childbirth.
- Engaging birth with your spouse in a way that strengthens your marriage.
- Leaving a legacy for your children with regard to pregnancy and birth.
- Surrendering idols concerning birth under the headship of Christ.

I am also very blessed and excited to share many different personal testimonies of like-minded mothers who have been blessed in one way or another in pregnancy and birth. My hope is that these testimonies will be an inspiration and encouragement, as well as impress upon you a thirst and hunger to seek God and His vision for your unique childbirth. May you be inspired with a new vision for the endless possibilities of what God may want to reveal through your birth.

Redeeming childbirth is not something we can do; it is something the Lord wants to do. We just need to surrender to Him. It will look different for everyone as we are all unique women on our unique journeys with the Lord, but we can all purpose to glorify Him through giving birth.

Let me share my prayer for you as you journey with me through a redeeming childbirth-

Jesus I thank you for the blessing of children and for the ability to partner with you to bring forth life. Thank you for my sisters who so deeply desire to glorify you during labor and birth. May you teach us all to trust you more and to love one another without judgement. May You be glorified and the church be unified. Lord, use this season during pregnancy to prepare my sisters for motherhood. Help us to accept our duties and responsibilities as Christian women in this day and age graciously. Help us to speak in love and build one another up. Lord, thank You for this privilege to serve You and honor You for what You have done for us. Thank you for blessing me with this message and providing the time and words to share all that is here. May You bless these women, their families, and may they have God-glorifying stories and testimonies to share in the future. To You be the glory forever and ever, Amen.

For further study while reading visit RedeemingChildbirth.com for a FREE download of *Reflective Journaling Questions* and Reader Only Downloads {code: Unity-in-Christ}

Part I

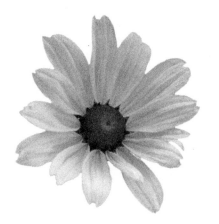

Every Woman has Her Story

Every woman has her story, but many do not feel the freedom to share it. A woman's journey to motherhood is an intimate one; her labor and birth experience have helped to mold who she has become today. This pilgrimage was for many thousands of years a catalyst to a common bond among women. It is a drastically different story today. But every woman still has her story and it is one worth telling, worth sharing, worth writing.

As a young mom, I remember gathering with other young moms at church for our monthly Moms of Preschoolers meeting. The easy get to know ya table talk usually started the same: birth stories. Every woman had a different story to tell . . . and women are much more eager to share their stories than they were even a generation ago.

My first born, Kelsey, was just six weeks old, so naturally the conversation was centered around babies and birthing experiences. I was seated at a table with four or five more experienced moms who had one to three children each. Since I was the first of my family and friends to get married and have a baby, I was excited to glean advice and eager to meet new friends and like-minded women.

The women in the group were really nice and it was apparent we all shared our love for Jesus in common. However, when it came to our birth experiences, they all seemed to be like-minded, complaining and comparing their horror stories with one another, I felt like an outcast. I became very quiet and shy and was afraid to share my positive experience for fear of making them feel bad or coming across as judgmental. I didn't want to make a bad first impression in the group and was overly concerned with what people thought of me.

Why would I make them feel bad? Because I had been so blessed with an amazing labor and birth. God had redeemed my childbirth experience by drawing me to closer and tenderly providing all I needed to birth my firstborn baby. I felt Him personally enriching and rewarding my laboring and birth. At this point, all of my most intimate personal relationships—with my husband, mother, newborn baby, and most of all with Christ—were strengthened and enriched. After my first birth, I felt I could conquer the world! I felt confident in the way God had made me as a woman and gladly pursued embracing that. I was still a first-time mother, learning everything along the way as most, but I had put a ton of personal responsibility into getting ready, and I felt God had blessed my efforts.

As the stories went around the table, I grew quiet—thinking and praying, wanting to share with them how amazing my experience truly was. I did not want to gloat, but had a deep desire to share with them a different God-glorifying perspective, in hope that they would receive transformed heart-attitudes from the Lord. I knew God wanted to minister to them and strengthen them just as much as He had me. God loves and cares for all his daughters the same . . . I only sought to let God be in control. Something we all try to do as Christians in EVERY area of our lives. Why not in childbirth?

I was about ready to burst with information, details, and emotional passion. Then my fear set in. People-pleasing fears consumed my thoughts as the stories continued around the table. Eagerly listening, waiting for someone to be the leader and say: "I am sorry you all had such terrible experiences, but may I offer hope? It does not have to be that way." As I listened to their stories, no one had mentioned God. I felt the Lord whispering to me, "Angie, please tell these women what I AM, who I AM, what I CAN do, and what I DID do."

It was now my turn . . . my hands were sweating . . . I was incredibly nervous. I began to share how I had a great birth. Timid, yet really desiring to honor God, I simply shared I had an amazing experience. Immediately, one woman spoke up with authority, "You got lucky. She's your first right?" Then another woman, who had delivered naturally, looked at me shocked and discriminately said, "You must have had an epidural." She was implying that she was better than us for having done it naturally, and that a natural birth without drugs to numb the pain could not have been a good experience, therefore, I MUST have not done it naturally.

Intimidated, I almost shrank back and said something like, "You are probably right," but my conviction after experiencing the Lord in such an intimate way would not allow me to believe what she was saying. But out of fear of them judging me, I muted my testimony of birth with God and only said, "No, I had a water birth." They all looked at me like I was an alien. Then one of them said, "So you chose to have a natural birth . . . it didn't just happen because your labor progressed too fast."

Out of respect, I shared with them a little of Kelsey's birth story. Now I am gratefully honored to share the whole experience with you here.

Kelsey's Birth Story

On the morning of her due date, I awoke around 6:30 a.m. after a great night's sleep. I went to the bathroom, lost my mucus plug, hopped in the shower, and began having strong contractions. So far the birthing process was going pretty predictably, according to everything I had read and prepared for. We planned to have our first baby at the local hospital, but I tried to focus and let my body do what I knew it was made to do as much as possible before heading there. Once we left, we called Waterbirth International to meet us at the hospital. We had planned to have a water birth, but the hospital we went to didn't have a birthing tub, so we brought our own. When we arrived, the doctor working our shift immediately tried to convince us we needed a caesarean. He said, "We think your baby is about nine pounds and since this is your first baby, she probably won't fit through your birth canal." That was when my husband kicked into his advocate and leader role. He spoke kindly to the doctor, but with authority as my protector. He handed the doctor our typewritten birth plan, and told the doctor if he didn't want to participate, to find someone else on staff to be on our team.

Just as he left, midwife and water-birth advocate Barbara Harper arrived with our birth tub and another midwife she was training. She asked if she could stay to train her midwife, which I felt was from the Lord, so, of course, I agreed. Just then, the on-staff midwife, Jane, and nurse Sammie (both Christians) entered the room. Even though water birth was not a hospital "cleared" alternative, Jane had always wanted to be a part of a water birth; so thankfully, she let us continue as planned, with the door locked. Barbara was such a blessing in my life that day. She taught me how to labor gracefully and she coached my husband on how to labor with me. He was in the birthing tub with me, praying over me, massaging me, and worshipping with me.

My mother, Vicki, was also a blessing to have there as she comforted, prayed, filled me up with words of affirmation and encouragement, and got in my face to help me focus. She believed in me, had faith that I could do this, that my body was made to do this. That was powerful for me as I pursued mental strength. Ultimately though, it was my relationship with the Lord that was my strength.

God was present with me there. He was strengthening my marriage, bonding my husband and me in such a deep way. We had to be a team. Isaac knew me well enough to know how I needed to be physically encouraged. Some women may not want anyone touching them, others may need their husbands to rub or kiss them. I needed different physical connections at different times in my laboring. It was essential for us to be able to communicate verbally and non-verbally in ways that strengthened our marriage. God was so good to allow us to experience birthing like this.

As I labored, I sang and talked to my baby. I couldn't wait to have her in my arms. In those moments when the contractions were so intense and seemingly unbearable, I leaned on my husband who was my rock.

He shared his strength with me as he spoke words of confidence and encouragement. He was always right by my side, going through each contraction with me. There were moments when I was floating on my back, with my head on his shoulder and nose tucked into his neck, I thought, "I can't do this. The pain is too intense and the baby isn't even crowning yet."

The he would whisper to me, "You are doing amazing Ang, I am so proud of you." He would pray for Jesus to give me rest, to be my strength, to help the baby come out soon. In those moments, our marriage was strengthened. He had confidence I could have this baby naturally; he believed in me. That empowered me.

Every song that played ministered to my soul. I could sense the presence of the Lord and His protection over me. Isaac held my pelvis under the water so that the baby's face would remain under the water as I was pushing. We experienced teamwork at its finest as he rocked me back and forth or held me still when I needed it.

As I labored in the water and sang songs of deliverance to my savior, the Lord brought to my mind thoughts of baptism and salvation of His people. Stories of the Lord's deliverance through water kept coming to the front of my mind.

Baptism had been a reoccurring theme the Lord had impressed upon me in my Bible studies. While I was pregnant my husband and I had been meeting with a mentor studying the topic, and as a youth pastor intern I had just led a study on the Hebrews' exodus from Egypt. God, in His goodness, protected Moses and his life was saved as he was sent down the river in a basket. God used the water to lead Moses to the Egyptian princess, who would adopt him as her own. One of the other ways God saved (delivered) the Israelites was through the parting of the Red Sea. As my birth progressed and I entered into the third stage of labor, known as transition, one of the songs on the CD reminded me of the works of the Lord through water. How He was sanctifying Jonah in the belly of the whale, teaching him through his experience of almost drowning in the sea and then sending a big fish to save him. Once he was ready, God released him and delivered him from the mouth of the whale. After having been refined in the whale, Jonah was willing to obey God. All of these stories rushed through my head as I focused on my deliverer, Jesus. I was so focused on these things above, on the truths from the Word of God, that it distracted me from focusing on the pain, though I still felt it. The Lord was about to deliver me, just as He had done for so many who had gone before me. When the hospital midwife asked to monitor our baby's heart rate and I had to stand for just even a moment, the pain seemed to triple. But the moment I sank back down into the water, I felt immediate relief. I felt as though the Lord was saving or rescuing me from my pain with the water. As I focused on this saving grace internally, though unable to share my thoughts with anyone around me, I found the Lord speaking intimately to me. He reminded me of how He was there with baby Moses, the Hebrew people, and Jonah when they needed to be delivered, and He was with me now.

Then as my daughter crowned, the midwife asked me if I wanted to catch her.

Surprised and delighted, I watched with a mirror, reaching down to embrace my daughter for the first time. Tucking my fingers under Kelsey's little arms, I turned her, while pushing. The Lord helped me push her out as I sang the last phrase of the song she was born to, "Someday." God had delivered me from the pain; He delivered my baby from the tight home she had outgrown. Birth was painful, but He delivered her out of me, and in turn I had no more pain. He set her free. I cried as I embraced the full reality that the Lord had blessed me; He had been there with me all the way. He had set me free, set her free that day.

The imagery that Jesus suffered to set me free from my sin, to set my daughter free from her sin, was so much more meaningful that day. I was overwhelmed by the presence of my babe in my arms, healthy and peaceful, but I was also overwhelmed by the presence of the Lord, my savior and deliverer. The fact that He had come with me to a tiny room at the end of the hall in a local hospital, to meet me there, to guide me, strengthen me, and make Himself known to me and to everyone in the room in such a way, made me fall in love with Him even more.

The lyrics were so perfect for delivering a baby under water . . . the song was chosen by God to be played at that moment. I felt His presence as I pushed her eight-pound, five-ounce body from mine. I felt a rush emotion flood my senses as I cleaned her off in the water allowing her to gently adapt to her surroundings for a brief second. The moment I embraced her to my bosom, I felt His presence. I experienced this sense of confidence in Him and faith in how He had created all of us for such moments as these. My husband Isaac and I were face to face with our baby girl for the first time. We were in awe of God, His gift to us in her.

"Someday"
(Set the Children Free)
Kelsey's Song from
"My Utmost for His Highest: The Covenant"
By Michael W. Smith

"The longing for the healing to come
Someday no more dark, aching nights . . .
Sometimes there's a joy in the pain...
Someday I will make all things whole
I promise to set the children free."

Isaac cut the umbilical cord and then spoke tenderly to her and she opened her eyes to the sound of her daddy's voice. We held her there in the birthing tub for a while. She was born gently; she was alert and attentive, calm and peaceful. As I nursed, we laughed, we cried, we prayed. She was born truly beautifully.

Her birth was an awesome experience on so many levels. Birth is the one time in a woman's life when she can count on the fact she will be challenged physically, verbally, mentally, emotionally, and spiritually, all simultaneously. Knowing this, expecting this reality, I prepared my heart by being in the Word. I prepared myself to involve God, let Him be the God who truly is omniscient (all knowing), omnipotent (all powerful), omnipresent (everywhere). The Deliverer, the Comforter, the Encourager/ Counselor (Holy Spirit), I let Him be my strength, and I wanted to praise Him for it.

Immediately after giving birth to Kelsey, I remember my husband asking me, "How do you feel, babe?" My reply was, "Like I was made to do this! I feel great!"

I was experiencing the adrenaline our bodies produce after natural childbirth. It was such a gift from God to be awake, aware, and soaking in every moment of enjoying our new blessing, without weariness. I stayed up cuddling her, nursing her, cherishing her with my husband. Listening to God's sweet whispers, I journaled the entire experience, to encourage and mentor my daughter when the time comes.

As I sat around the table with these other young moms, I shared how I had experienced God in my labor and water birth. I recounted how my daughter was born fairly quickly in five and a half hours, that I was able to deliver her myself, and how amazing it was for my husband and me, and strengthened my relationship with the Lord. I told them it was one of the best experiences in my life; nothing like it. Their eyes glazed and I felt so alone all of a sudden. I felt judged, while in a church moms' group, for having had a good birth and for having chosen to have a natural birth. My fears quickly became a reality after I finished my short story. Then the negative comments began: "Well you got lucky, she was your first . . . just you wait." "How long was your labor? Oh, five hours? Just wait until you get one that's twenty hours." As you can imagine, I felt like an outcast. I felt alone, like no one there understood or could relate to the intimacy I had experienced with my husband, my baby, and my Lord. Inside a war of emotions was raging. I didn't know if I should cry for release of that nauseating gut feeling you get when you feel so judged or when God is being misrepresented. Or if I should speak out in truth, confidentially sharing what spiritual milestone childbirth had been. Inside, a battle was raging. I was confused and scared . . . were they telling the truth? Was I really just lucky? Or was my experience truly a blessing from the Lord? Was He trying to teach me something that was intended for others as well? Had I experienced the way God intended childbirth to be approached? I just wanted to encourage these women that God wants to be a part of every area of our lives, even our births, but I wasn't ready.

As the years passed and the Lord continued to bless our family with more children (six so far), I felt even more isolated. I wanted so badly to share with women that God could redeem their childbirth. That it doesn't have to be an event in our lives that we fear or try to avoid. It is an experience we can look forward to with great anticipation. I wanted to tell them how He had redeemed mine, as a testimony to His grace and mercy, and that He also wants to do that for them.

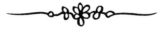

What Is the Gap?

Within the Christian community, there are two ditches on either side of the road, and they form the gap. On one side you have the women in the church who are labeled as extreme. They are accused of being judgmental women who stubbornly hold to the perspective that home births are spiritually superior; some might even say, "You must not be a strong Christian unless you have a home birth." On the opposing side you have the women who don't look much different than the rest of today's culture. They view pregnancy and birth as a burden to be avoided, even an ailment. They may not say it, but they focus on the limitations that come with pregnancy and fear birth more than the blessings. Unfortunately, the judgment is thick and destructive on both sides. While one group is stubbornly holding to the perspective that only home births can be spiritual, the opposing side holds tightly to their opinion that voluntarily experiencing pain in natural childbirth when they don't have to is crazy.

May I call out this battle within the church among women? Ladies, why the disunity? There is a gap between the two extremes within the Christian faith where different views and potholes can converge.

Redeeming Childbirth does not condemn anyone, but exhorts all women to seek God in all things, including pregnancy and childbirth. I believe God wants us to shed light on the lies we as women have grown to believe, the lies that have seeped into the church and caused this friction. Stand in the gap with me! Pursue God, pursue truth, and filter all things through the Word of God, including advice from doctors, midwives, books, friends, and even family members. If you have received Christ and call yourself a follower, then you need to invite God to be a part of your whole life, not just compartments of it. We need Jesus to lead us, change us, mold us, transform us, and heal us. When He redeemed us and saved us from our sin, the price was paid once and for all so that in Him we can have eternal life.

Before we are called to be with Him in heaven, we have the blessing and gift of the presence of the Holy Spirit to guide us and comfort us. We need to pursue Jesus and invite Him to be an active part of our everyday lives. In our arrogance to work within our own strength, we waste it pursuing emptiness, when we could be experiencing the fullness of His power in our weakness.

If we claim home births are the most spiritual, wouldn't that be putting God in a box? God is everywhere and He wants to be invited everywhere, birth centers and hospitals included. However, if we are Christians and we are to engage the culture but clearly look different from it, why has there been an adoption of secular thinking within the church? Why this entitlement attitude of not deserving to feel pain? Why are we, as a church, accepting secular and new age perspectives on childbirth? Why are the majority of Christians' views on childbirth based on fear?

Something Is Missing in Today's Christian Culture

We are a blessed nation and people, but we need perspective. The prosperity we enjoy has led to an entitlement mentality that has crept into our Christian homes and churches. This attitude of selfish indulgence breeds ideas in us that we shouldn't have to experience hardships or trials in life. We'll go to great lengths to avoid the consequences of our choices and unwittingly only delay God's law of sowing and reaping. Sadly, by dodging rather than engaging these challenges, we cripple ourselves because we fail to learn this life lesson of cause and effect. This failure to grow and learn makes us less prepared to tackle the bigger trials in life that will undoubtedly come.

God says in Romans 5:4, "More than that we rejoice in our sufferings, knowing that suffering produces endurance, and endurance produces character, and character produces hope, and hope does not put us to shame, because God's love has been poured into our hearts through the Holy Spirit who has been given to us."

The blessing of growth comes from persevering through the trial, through experiencing the suffering. As Christians, we need to prepare for what the Lord has planned for our lives. He allows us to experience pain and trials to make us stronger. If we avoid our opportunities for growth in the process, leaning on Him, growing in Him, experiencing His promises fulfilled and the depth of conviction that grows within our souls, we could potentially be less prepared later in life. It is easy to praise Him during good times, but more challenging to praise and worship Him while we are undergoing pain.

We have got to stand up against the culture's message. We need to quit being concerned with following the crowd and being so politically correct that we sacrifice just speaking truth. We don't need to do what everyone else is doing-- popping a pill to numb the pain and avoid reality—because then we miss out on the blessings and growth God has planned for us.

Instead we should embrace life with all its challenges, trials, pains, and disappointments. We trust and follow God as our shepherd who leads us, our father who protects us. We need to quit getting in the way and allow God to be who He is and do what He does best. Let Him be glorified. Allow Him to do miracles. Allow Him to be obvious to people. Sometimes, we need to resolve to be weak and human, and let Him be God. We need to intentionally let Him penetrate our everyday lives.

Pregnancy is the time God has gifted us with to prepare us for birth and motherhood. Our labor of love begins in pregnancy; through the intensity of childbirth we can become better prepared for a lifetime of laboring in love for our children. It is the beginning of a journey for a woman growing into motherhood. *Redeeming Childbirth* is the outcry for Christian women to stand up and purposefully choose to give God their pregnancies and birth experiences in whatever form they see it as. Invite Him to be involved; embrace the beautiful design of womanhood God has created and believe He is enough and has designed your body to bring forth life.

This is an opportunity to train our hearts, minds, and souls to surrender all to God. As a parent, you have to surrender control a lot. Giving God your birth is just one opportunity in life out of many to surrender all to the Lord. This is something we, as parents, need to practice in order for our muscle of surrendering to be fit to give Him back the blessings He gives us in our children. This is a practice worth striving for in every area of our lives.

Together, let's shine Jesus' light on those two ditches on either side of the road and all the potholes in between. Together let's hold one another accountable to serve the only God who deserves our praise and adoration. Let us not make idols out of things or people that will distract us from seeking Him. When we are fearful or being tested, let's embrace life and its challenges. We need to understand that God has allowed us to walk through this life with open hearts and that fear does not come from Him. Then we can proactively choose to have teachable hearts, open to divine refinement about life, others, Him, and ourselves. Learning and growing through seasons of suffering can transform an otherwise painful experience into a spiritual milestone.

Ultimately, as Christians we need to seek unity on this issue of birth—unity with respect. We need to respect the truth that every woman is on her own spiritual journey with the Lord. In regard to where the birth takes place—home, hospital, or birth center—we need to have grace enough to allow people to be on their own journeys and understand that having a baby in one place or another doesn't necessarily determine where their faith lies. Judging is never fulfilling. What is fulfilling though, is women speaking truth and encouraging other women. What is fulfilling is older, more experienced women sharing their ideas and visions with younger women to give hope, permission to dream, and a bridge to Jesus where He can guide them in their decision-making. We need unity within families,

ITS NOT ABOUT HOW YOU HAVE THE BABY BUT MAKING SURE
GOD IS AT THE CENTLE OF IT ALL.

where mothers, daughters, and sisters are strong enough to be honest about each other's lives and share these intimate moments together.

We can bridge this gap among women in the church if we focus on Christ and His deep desire to be present in all of our lives, including childbirth. Older women should teach that Christ can be a part of a woman's birth anywhere and under any circumstances. The focus needs to move off of where the baby's birth happens, to how we purposefully include Jesus to be a part of it. If you are focused on Jesus and what He wants for your birth, the where and how will fall into place.

I believe Christ Himself can redeem this gap. He can bridge it if we focus on Him. He wants unity among His people, His family. This topic is very sensitive and intimate, one I believe God wants to see His daughters agree on. We may have variations in our birth experiences, as long as there is unity in the Spirit. He wants women to rise up and behold His glory in childbirth. He simply wants to be invited!

There are clearly times when women experience emergencies in birth. That being said, *Redeeming Childbirth* has a special chapter regarding those situations. For now, let's focus on inviting Jesus into our births and strive to let Him teach us and control our birthing experiences. Allow Him to challenge us and grow us. I believe His desire isn't to see all Christians having homebirths, but to be invited to the experience. He wants every one of His daughters to include Him in every experience of their lives.

A Special Note to First Time Moms

Inviting Jesus into your birth experience isn't complicated. If you have given Jesus your heart, given Him your life, then asking Him to lead your every decision in regard to your birth and care of your baby is the next step. Seeking Him, ask Him to go before you and prepare you throughout your pregnancy for motherhood. In prayer, invite Him to walk through this entire journey with you.

Prayer Journal Entry April 2000
Lord, I am in awe of the amazing gift You have blessed me with. I am expecting my first baby and feel so inadequate to be blessed with this great privilege to raise this child You have made inside my womb. I am overwhelmed and unsure of my abilities. I am relying on You and need more of You. I am sick, I am tired, I am scared, and yet I am so thankful. Jesus, thank You for giving me just enough physical strength when I need it, but please heal me from this excessive morning sickness. Help me not to be scared. Give me peace and take my anxiety away. Help me have self-control over my emotions. I give my life, my baby, my marriage, everything to You, Lord. Please use me to glorify You. I want more than anything to be used by You. Refine me and make me more like You. Help me stay positive and focused on You when I don't feel well. Help me not to worry, but to cast my fears on You. Please bring friends into my life who can encourage me and whom I can encourage and be real with. I feel so alone sometimes Lord. Lord, be my all in all, my best friend. Be more than enough for me, Lord. ~Ang

Redeeming the Division

Creating an Atmosphere of Acceptance and Love in the Church

The division among women in the church on this hot topic of labor and delivery is the big pink elephant in the room. Every woman knows it's there. They all take sides and yet no one ever speaks out on it. The sisters are in sin. Bonded by the blood of their Father, but divided by the lies of the enemy, women in the church today have been deceived. This deception is clever on their enemy's part, for he knows the pride of man all too well.

The Savior, Jesus Christ, watches and grieves. His heart grieves for the pain this division causes. Why don't they just recognize the enemy has deceived them yet again? Not only does this division create disunity among sisters in the Body of believers but also between every woman and their Lord. Sin, it creeps in so slowly, we don't even see it. We justify our intentions and continue letting the divide grow farther and wider among us.

Our God wants us, His daughters, to be united. He does not want us divided by things that are not eternal. 1 Timothy 2:15 says, "But women will be saved through childbearing—if they continue in faith, love and holiness with propriety." Childbearing is very dear to our Father's heart as you will discover in the coming chapters. Because it is so close to our

Father's heart, I am compelled to speak out on this secretive, deceptive divide among women in the church today.

We need healing, we need unity, we need Jesus to redeem childbirth in the church today. When we find common ground in Christ and choose to focus on glorifying Him on this topic of childbearing, acknowledging and respecting that we are all on our own spiritual journeys, then we can receive His redeeming work in the church at large with regard to childbirth.

In the spirit of unity, let us come together under one head—which is Christ—to be a better example of Christ's love for the world. Let's approach birth from a different perspective. Let's rise up, Church, unified, and seek to embrace God's design of "womb-man." Let's surrender to the Lord and receive His blessing that is found in the mission of birth and the gift of children. Let's uplift one another, not judge. Let's pray together for the Lord to convict our hearts in areas where we have been judgmental and ugly. Let's ask God to help us trust that He made our bodies for the purpose of bringing forth life, and ask Him to renew our minds and our perspectives on pregnancy, birth, pain, and the gift of motherhood. Let's rise up and make a difference in this next generation together. Let's lead together, in love and unity, toward a movement of women in the church purposing to invite Jesus into all areas, events, and experiences in our lives. We are all sisters in this body. Let's work together and embrace that we share this amazing blessing that is the gift of childbirth.

I believe God's desire for women in the church is to become more intentional in our relationships and in each season of life. So let's embark on this journey of seeking what His Word teaches about childbirth and examine the many different ways in which we can glorify Him in unity. We are all on the same team, Team Jesus, so let's support and encourage one another while we are here in this life. It is short and we are here for many reasons, one of which is to glorify Him with our lives. May it be a sweet offering to Him who has redeemed us.

So are you with me?

Choosing to be a part of this movement within the church, a movement of women recognizing their God-given influence, in setting the culture of the church, means we stop caring about what others think of us and speak truth in love, for the glory of God. When a sister in the Lord shares a bad birth experience, we should take the time to get to know her, care for her, help her to deal with any trauma, and gently share with her the truth. We need to help her overcome any fear caused by her birth experience. Provide a healthy place for her to share her story, without it traumatizing other young birthing mothers, by having her over for tea to talk. Explain to her how harmful it could be for other pregnant women to hear her skewed perspective on birth. Try to help her focus on anything good she could have learned from this experience. Oftentimes women who focus on their bad experiences only need someone to ask them what they learned, or what God did through their experiences, to help them heal and gain fresh perspectives.

Part II

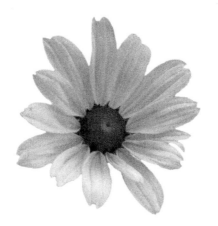

Redeeming Childbirth

———— ❧❧❧ ————

What do you think of when you think of the word redeemed?

For many believers, the answer to this question is more than a definition or description of what it means to "redeem" something. For many the word redeem holds a personal and spiritual connotation.

What does it mean to REDEEM?[1]

To Redeem:[2]

1. To purchase back; to ransom; to liberate or rescue from captivity or bondage, or from any obligation or liability to suffer or to be forfeited, by paying an equivalent; as, to redeem prisoners . . .
2. To repurchase what has been sold; to regain possession of a thing alienated, by repaying the value of it to the possessor.
3. To rescue; to recover; to deliver from.
4. To compensate, to make amends for.
5. To free by making atonement.
6. To pay the penalty of.
7. To save.
8. To perform what has been promised.

---

9. In law, to recall an estate, or to obtain the right to re-enter upon a mortgaged estate by paying to the mortgage his principle, interest and expenses or costs.

10. "In theology, to rescue and deliver from the bondage of sin and the penalties of God's violated law, by obedience and suffering in the place of the sinner, or by doing and suffering that which is accepted in lieu of the sinner's obedience. Christ hath redeemed us from the curse of the law, being made a curse for us. Gal. Iii. Tit.ii"

What is a REDEEMER?

A redeemer is 1) One who redeems or ransoms; or 2) The Savior of the world, Jesus Christ.

What is the vision and mission behind Redeeming Childbirth?

God deeply desires for us all to know Him and His redeeming power in every area of our lives. As I have mentioned before, the division among the women of God on this topic of childbirth is in grave need of being redeemed. For too long, we as a church have allowed our enemy to divide our team and make us less effective for the kingdom of God. What once used to be a strong common bond among women, now divides. I believe God wants to redeem that.

Secondly, God desires to redeem your personal childbirth experience. Whether you have experienced a traumatic birth already and you are need of healing in your heart, soul and mind, or you are about to give birth for the first time—God wants you to experience His presence and know Him more intimately.

This book was written to first and foremost glorify the Lord—for what He has done and is doing in countless women's lives. God wants a deep relationship with each and every one of His daughters. You can have that deep relationship with Him regardless of how you birth your babies, but He wants to be invited to experience this special event with you.

The Lord has gifted us with the privilege to bring forth man, and even though we still feel the consequences of the curse in the form of pain in childbearing, He nevertheless desires to bless us, deliver us, and grow our relationships to be more reconciled to Him.

I think every woman in the midst of labor would agree there is a deep desire at one point or another to cry out for someone to relieve or save her from the pain. God however, is often not the One asked. But we are in need of saving. We are in need of deliverance, both eternally and during childbirth, and God is the only One who can save us—who can redeem our birth experiences and pain.

Childbirth, as well as many other intimate issues among women in the church is in need of being redeemed. We have already discussed the division that exists among women on this topic and the need to unify and educate them to teach women to intentionally glorify God in how they approach pregnancy, childbirth, and motherhood. I believe that God has so much to offer each and every one of us—His beloved daughters—and we have much to gain from His presence in our journeys. We cannot redeem our own childbirths, but we can ask Jesus Christ to.

We as women need to approach birth with the same goal in mind: to glorify and be obedient to our Lord's call on our lives. Our births do NOT need to look the same, but we as the Church should look different than the world in how we view, approach and engage pregnancy and childbirth. We need to humbly come to our Father in submission to His will for our lives and encourage others to do the same, without judgment. The Lord desires to bring unity among women. Though our births may look different, the Lord can redeem the division if we are all pursuing to seek Him and His will for our births, and if we can choose to not look at circumstances but rejoice for what good God is doing and has done in one another's lives through our birth experiences.

We are all in need of a redeemer; we cannot EARN our salvation. Jesus is that redeemer, who came to save us from our sins. He wants to redeem all the moments in our lives, not just the Sunday mornings. He wants to redeem our marriages, our families, our relationships, and He also wants to redeem the unsaved people in our lives. He came to redeem the world. God deeply desires to redeem our trials, our sufferings, and our pain. Jesus wants to redeem our experiences in life as well, and purposes to bring glory to the Kingdom of God.

We, as a society, have compartmentalized birth to institutions and in doing so we have consequentially compartmentalized Jesus out of birth.

I am not an advocating for or against hospital births here. What I am advocating is for Christ to be allowed back into the experience. And not only should He be allowed back into the experience, but He should be given supreme authority. In most cases, when anything is institutionalized, the truth to be found is that God is OFTEN not welcome. It is not that He is not there … it is that He is not often acknowledged or invited. This needs to change. Any woman can give birth in a hospital and experience the Lord's presence. It is not where the baby is born that marks a birth as redeemed. It is the act of surrendering our agendas to the Lord, seeking His will for our childbirth, and then experiencing His presence working in us, through us, and around us that makes it a redemptive milestone in one's life.

Compartmentalizing Jesus is a problem that reaches far beyond childbirth. As Christians, we need to be careful and examine how we live our lives and make our decisions. Do we go to God with every decision? Do we seek His wisdom before we make choices? Or do we act in our own selfish, sinful nature, making decisions based on how we feel, what we fear, or what the culture tells us we should do?

The Cure for Compartmentalizing Jesus

In order for the Lord to redeem our experiences, we need to deliver them into His hands. We need to choose to hand over experiences such as holidays that no longer focus on Him (Easter, Christmas, Reformation Day); and weddings, birthdays, and even mundane experiences like doing dishes and gardening. He is in it all and we seem to take Him for granted. We sometimes forget to be thankful for having loads of laundry to fold because they represent all the bodies that wear them. To a certain degree, we as Christians have accidentally allowed our God to become alienated from our daily routines, holidays, and life experiences, but especially childbirth.

The only cure for compartmentalizing Jesus is to live the conviction that Jesus is life. To live the conviction that your contribution to be made on earth is to intentionally glorify Him in all you do, to integrate your faith in Him and the wisdom of His Word into your daily experiences. We need more of Jesus in every area of our lives. This process is going to have to be intentional!

Let's reclaim our experiences and actively pursue acknowledging God in all things, being our all in all. Let's chose to be vulnerable and let God show us His redeeming power in our experiences, including childbirth.

As Jesus' ambassadors we have the privilege of shining for Him, actively working as servants to the cross, proclaiming His truth to all. He uses us to bring His Word and love to those in our lives, to introduce Him to them, so that they too might be saved. We shine our light by allowing God to express His power in and through our lives. Proclaiming His good works through personal testimony is one of the most powerful tools of evangelism.

Allowing God's presence during childbirth glorifies Him. He takes what can be an exciting but painful experience and converts it into an experience that has massive spiritual significance in our lives and the lives of those we share it with. The curse brought forth a type of bondage and physical commitment. Jesus wants to rescue us from that bondage and prepare us through the physical commitment. We still have pain in birth today, but if we ask Him to be present and to be glorified, He will redeem our experience and bless us in so many ways. It will not be an experience dreaded, but rather one that is a milestone in our spiritual lives.

On a broader viewpoint, childbirth is in need of being redeemed by God in regard to all of the false teachings, worldly perspectives, and secular and new age influences. We women of the body of Christ need to include God in our births. We need to invite Him and experience His presence. We need to allow Him to transform the church's view of childbirth into one that reflects biblical truth. This transformation starts in our hearts, and from there we can go forth, encouraging young women in the church, teaching them of God's truths and His power. God desires so badly for your birth to be a redemptive experience, where you grow in your relationship with Him richly and deeply. And He doesn't want it to only benefit you, but wants you to share with others how you have been blessed so they can have vision for what God has in store for them.

Do you see how beautiful this can be for the church? Women united in speaking truth, ministering to one another, loving one another, and bonding together because of their common faith in the salvation of Christ and deep connection that comes from experiencing His grace in birth. Imagine the ways we could build one another up as we share His stories with other women and our children. As of now, birth divides women more than it brings them together. Anything that brings disunity grieves the heart of our Father in heaven. Let Him be the glue that closes this division and brings unity among women in love, through truth and acceptance.

Biblically, it is clear the Lord disciplined all of His daughters with pain in childbearing. Why do we avoid experiencing this discipline? Scripture tells us as followers of Christ, "For the moment all discipline seems painful rather than pleasant, but later it yields the peaceful fruit of righteousness to those who have been trained by it," (Hebrews 12:11). Why do we have such hardened hearts toward reproof, correction, and discipline when they are clearly for our good and make us more holy?

Could it be that we were not raised to be thankful and to acknowledge that it was meant for our growth?

Or has the culture around us influenced our thinking and our reactions so much we cannot comprehend why anyone would experience pain when they have a choice not to? Does a child have a choice to be disciplined after being disobedient or defiant? Does an adult who commits a crime and is caught have the choice to walk away from his punishment? Why do we pursue avoiding a discipline that was meant for our potential good? We are fighting an internal battle in which our physical self wants to have control over an experience that requires surrender in spirit, mind, and body under God's headship and authority. What we don't realize is we were not intended to live apart from God. We attempt to live our lives without Him and fail more often than not and end up frustrated.

Isn't this the oppression of the curse, you might ask? I recognize this is a hard message to embrace. It has been for me as I prepared my heart to be even more refined with each successive childbirth. But I share this with you, because once you choose to surrender fully under the headship of the Lord, you begin living in the freedom of the grace that Jesus brings. You begin to view the pain, not as a burden or a curse, but as beautiful. It is a beautiful pain because of the spiritual, mental, and emotional growth you will experience as you embrace it, in Christ who strengthens you.

I love you, my sisters in Christ. When a woman fully surrenders her birth to Christ and seeks to allow Him to redeem it, it will look different for every woman. Just as I said before, we are all on our own beautiful spiritual journey. If you are not in a place ready to implement all that *Redeeming Childbirth* can offer that is fine. God just wants to grow you. For some, it may look like baby steps, and for others it will be an amazing transformation. Either way, the Lord loves us all equally. There is nothing we could ever do to make Him love us more. He just wants you to know all the ways in which He wants to bless you.

Today, the typical birth experience is not viewed as an experience to look forward to. Often childbirth is feared and avoided in one way or another. But Jesus wants to regain possession of our hearts in every area of our lives. We talk about how to incorporate God into your birth experience if you have an epidural in "What about an Emergency." I don't want you to be discouraged in thinking the only way to experience God in birth is through a natural birth. That is simply NOT true and I talk about that later in another chapter, but God can meet you in a very unique way in natural childbirth.

Let me share my heart with you for a moment. I have experienced something amazing with my Lord. Not because I am amazing, I am NOT. I really am ordinary. I simply have an extraordinary God. He is so gracious, merciful, and loving. This is hard for me to share with others, because, it is so intimate. Not just the act of childbirth, but also the blessing of intimacy I felt with my Lord.

When you are empty and ready to give up, and you are working hard, so hard, with no breaks, you can get to a place (that most don't experience with an epidural) where He is all you have left. And He is more than enough. As you are focused on Him and not on yourself, God takes something so many people view as primitive and unnecessary, making it beautiful and fruitful.

For me, as I watched my husband Isaac see me praying, worshiping, crying out to God, leaning on Him—strong not in myself, but clearly in Him—I noticed a renewed respect and admiration for me that I realized could never be thwarted. As I glanced over at my daughters, who were praying and laying their hands on my head and shoulders, I also noticed a true faith in their souls and a firm belief as they diligently prayed to God.

Once you finally hold your baby and realize it wasn't in your power but God's that helped you birth your baby, you will praise Him for what He has done personally in your life. Your childbirth can become a testimony of God's miraculous works.

What compels me to tell you this? Because for some reason, God has burdened my heart to tell you about the great things He has done in my births and many other's births. And to tell you He wants to meet you there too! He wants to go with you, to give you strength, to be your all-in-all. He wants to do something glorious and to be glorified.

The Lord wants you to recognize He is the One who delivers babies. He delivers you from the pain of birth once your child is in your arms. I find it ironic that when someone is birthing a baby the term used for it is "delivering" a baby. The person who catches the baby is called the one who delivered the baby. One of the definitions of deliverance is "the act of bringing forth children" (N. Webster's 1828 Dictionary). "To deliver" has many meanings: to rescue, to release from restraint, to save, to transfer into another's hand or power, "to disburden of a child" (referring to childbirth), to give up, and to surrender. The definition for deliverer is compelling in its own right as well:

Deliver [3]

1. To free; to release, as from restraint . . . to deliver one from captivity (such as the curse of pain in childbearing).
2. To rescue, or save.
3. To give, or transfer; to put into another's hand or power; to commit; to pass from one to another.
4. To surrender; to yield; to give up; to resign; as to deliver a fortress to an enemy.
5. To disburden a child.
6. To utter; to pronounce; to speak; to send forth in words; as, to deliver a sermon
7. To exert in motion.
8. To surrender or resign, to abandon to.

Jesus is our deliverer in birth. He brings forth life. He chooses when that baby will be born; we know not the hour, only He does. He is the one we can choose to transfer our pain to, to let Him take it and carry us. He can speak truth to us in this intimate experience. He alone rescues and delivers one from captivity. He wants His daughters to experience Him deeply in this way, consciously aware that He is in control and is the Deliverer. But we have a responsibility as well. We have to deliver or surrender our pain, our fears, our expectations, our childbirths, and ultimately our lives unto the Lord. We have to ask Him to deliver us.

We like to take control over the planning of our births, and it is okay to prepare and plan, but we need to submit those plans to the Lord.

We can actively choose to participate with God by inviting Him to redeem our childbirths in whichever way He chooses for us. Our God has made us unique and we are all on our own spiritual journeys, but we must make the choice to surrender our lives to Him in every area and be careful not to compartmentalize Jesus.

What does redeeming childbirth look like in practical terms?

For some it will be embracing natural childbirth. For others it will be embracing an emergency situation and allowing God to refine them through it. Some may experience Him in a new way by intentionally incorporating worship, song, meditative prayer, or collective prayer with a community of saints gathered together in their labor and birth. And to others, simply seeking first His kingdom may lead one to truly engage in opportunities for evangelism with care givers—whether in the hospital, birth center, or home. God can strengthen the bond between a husband and wife, a mother and daughter, between sisters and friends through the journey shared together. Bonding together in this spiritual way benefits everyone involved, creating a deeper spiritual intimacy in the family. Sometimes what God chooses to do in your heart or the hearts of others in your life through watching you prepare is what is redeeming.

There are so many ways in which God can redeem birth. The Lord loves us all and deeply desires deeper, more intimate relationships with us. More specifically, He wants to walk beside you through life, carry your burdens, protect you, and give you strength and guidance, but most of all He wants your whole heart and soul to be fully engaged with His Spirit. God, our Father, desires a deep relationship with all of His daughters— one with no boundaries. Walls cannot bind God and we constantly try to put limitations on what the Lord can do in our lives and through us—simply by refusing to surrender control.

Redeeming Childbirth is not a book just about natural birth, although there are many God-glorifying testimonies to what He has done in and through them. *Redeeming Childbirth* is more than just how you decide to birth your baby. It's about your intentions, your motives, your heart attitudes and your relationships. In this very special season in a woman's life when she is with child and preparing for motherhood, there are many opportunities for growth—in relationships as well as spiritually.

Have you ever heard the phrase, "Where your heart is, there your treasure will be"? In childbirth your attitude, convictions, and beliefs will be tested. If your heart is focused on glorifying the Lord in childbirth, that truth will be revealed and shine brightly to all who are witnesses it. Certain aspects of your heart can be reflected in your attitude toward pregnancy as well as how you labor. What you focus on when preparing for parenthood, how you react to pain and circumstances, how you treat others, how you view the birth process, how you view your body, your baby, your husband and your God (with regard to birth) all reflect heart attitudes (both good and bad), as well as potential areas of sin. This is exciting for one main reason—when we are honest with ourselves and choose to engage the truth within us, we can grow spiritually as we seek our Redeemer and allow Him to refine us. This is the sanctifying aspect of childbirth and motherhood—recognizing one's sin and selfishness and choosing to repent and allowing God to transform our hearts.

When we as women of God engage this challenge to grow and choose to believe in the Lord's promises, then we will have more open hearts toward submitting our will under His headship. Is Jesus the Lord of your whole life? Or the areas that are most comfortable? Is God or religion something we as a church compartmentalize out of birth?

These questions are at the heart of *Redeeming Childbirth*:

Do we Christians birth any different from those in the world who don't believe in the redeeming power of Jesus? Can nurses and doctors tell we are different by the way we birth? If we don't look different—why don't we? Aren't we supposed to be the light of the world?

God wants to redeem childbirth in general. We can glorify Him and show the world the true power of our God as we worship and praise Him throughout labor and childbirth.

We teach this concept to our youth when it comes to making decision—WWJD (what would Jesus do?)—but we often fail to ask ourselves this question with regard to major life decisions, circumstances, or life transitions such as pregnancy and childbirth. How would Jesus act? How would He respond to these circumstances (fear or faith)? Then we need to pursue following in His example—that should be our pursuit—to glorify our Lord by seeking to live righteously, honoring His name.

God does not have a cookie-cutter plan for any of our lives, let alone our births. But I think He does desire us all to "seek first the kingdom of God and his righteousness, and all these things will be added to you," (Matthew 6:33). God wants to bless us with all wisdom and knowledge, but those things will be given to us once we seek first His Kingdom. Our motives need to be righteous and for the glory of His Kingdom.

Childbirth is one of the beginning experiences that enter us into motherhood. Parenthood is a labor of love that never ends . . . I would encourage you to begin the journey of seeking Him as your main counselor and guide in this transition, now—in the beginning.

Inviting the Lord to redeem your childbirth begins by surrendering this journey and our wills to the Lord—it is giving it to Him, to let Him do with it what He wills. The beauty in this is that God has a personal relationship with each of us so His redeeming of our births will not look the same. He will custom-fit our birth stories if we submit them to Him.

Jesus can and wants to be the hero in your birth story. "Thus says the Lord, your Redeemer, who formed you from the womb; 'I am the Lord, who made all things, who alone stretched out the heavens, who spread the earth by myself,'" (Isaiah 44:24). He wants to liberate and rescue you from all bondage, including any emotional, mental, spiritual, and physical bondage you may have in your life. He can do that work in your life as you embrace and prepare for childbirth with Him. Prepare your heart, mind, soul, and body, and choose to pursue healing in all of those aspects through Christ Jesus in order to experience all God wants to bless you with in a redeemed birth experience. Jesus wants you to rely on Him and to deliver you from your pain when He delivers your baby. He is the redeemer. He is the deliverer.

In order for God to fully redeem childbirth we need to have teachable hearts open to viewing pregnancy, birth, and motherhood through a biblical lens that impresses upon us the importance of God's control over our lives. His works in each woman's heart will slowly refine the church. Just as He commanded the Israelites to "Remember these things, O Jacob, and Israel, for you are my servant; I formed you and you will not be forgotten by me. I have blotted out your transgressions like a cloud and your sins like a mist; return to me, for I have redeemed you," (Isaiah 44:21-22). Our fathers in the faith, Abraham and Jacob, were commanded to remember the things the Lord had done, how He had delivered them with a promise to redeem them by way of "blotting out their sins." He wants us to return to Him as fully surrendered servants.

We are to remember what Jesus has done for us—all of the instances when we experienced His faithfulness and redeeming power in our lives. When we experience His presence in childbirth, we should remember and pass on the legacy of faith through sharing our testimonies with others, as servants to the message of the cross. May we purposefully allow Him to refine us, teach us, and bless us. As sisters in Christ, may we come together to build one another up, encouraging one another so God may be glorified.

I hope you are empowered, and your belief that the Lord is alive and active today in His peoples' lives is strengthened. I pray as you read you would have a new vision and dare to dream of your perfect birth.

Pray with me

Lord I thank You for the gift of motherhood and how it challenges us to grow, no matter how we encounter it. I pray Lord, that this message reaches many mothers, even those who do not have a natural birth, and that they would feel Your presence. I pray they would not feel condemnation, but empowerment in seeking you in whatever journey you allow for them to walk through. Lord, we know guilt is not from You, and my heart is not to bring guilt. I pray my sisters would dare to dream. Dream of births where You are their focus and where their husbands are praying over them and engaged in the process of labor. I pray more than anything my sisters would feel empowered and excited for the births of their babies, and be brought to a place of confidence in You.

I also pray for the first-time mother who is reading this Lord. Please guide her in wisdom as she prepares and plans for this baby. May her focus be on seeking You. I pray for her marriage and the relationships in her life; I ask that a few strong women would come beside her as she prepares for motherhood, to teach her and pray for her. I pray for her to find like-minded sisters in the faith who want to spur one another on toward growth in You and delight in Your purposes and blessings.

Lastly, I pray we would all be open to learning about God and the simple yet amazing ways He can be a part of our everyday lives. May we all live for His glory, not our own, shining a light strong in the darkness, so we may go forth and make disciples of all nations, even where we are now. Thank You, Father, that You have redeemed us, and Your work was done on the cross. Thank You that we can live in freedom, here on earth and in the life to come. Give us the power of your Holy Spirit to overcome whatever comes our way. For You are the power and the glory forever and ever, Amen.

Birth is Bigger than My Belly

When planning for her wedding, a woman spends countless hours preparing every last detail, including the embossing type on the reception napkins. Our culture's focus on this momentous day influences ladies from a very young age to dream about our perfect day. As Christian women who grow up in a world that promotes "happy ever afters," I recognize we are tempted by all the hype of being the center of attention and get distracted from what is truly important in preparing for marriage. Similarly, the excitement and anticipation grows within the heart of the first-time mother when she finds out she is with child. With great excitement, a woman prepares her home for the addition to her family. She plans projects to finish before her baby is born, paints and decorates her baby's room. She researches diapers, carriers, strollers, and all the other gadgets our culture tells her are necessary. Some women go to birthing classes and read a book or two on what to expect in attempts to try to be prepared for the birth day. The mother-to-be works diligently at being as prepared as possible for the day she starts her journey of motherhood, hoping that being prepared will make her a better mother.

The reality is no cloth diaper or baby carrier is going to make you a better mommy. Just as young couples can find themselves wildly disappointed and shocked at the realities married life brings, so can a young couple bringing their baby home from the hospital.

Do you remember the saying, "Honey, the wedding day ain't the marriage?" I was told this little nugget of wisdom from a few older women when I was planning my wedding. What they meant was . . . be careful not to get caught up in the hype of the wedding day or things you think will make it perfect. Instead be wise to prepare for the long run of marriage, prepare spiritually, because that is what will get you through the hard times that are sure to come. So it is with preparing for the day of your child's birth.

Just as "the wedding day ain't your marriage," birth is bigger than your belly and your child's birth day ain't motherhood.

Conception and pregnancy are monumental primary experiences in motherhood and so is childbirth. Preparing for the experience of childbirth is wise, but what is the wisest thing to focus on: buying all the gadgets and nesting as they say, or preparing your relationships (with God, your husband, your mother, your friends, etc) for this new season in life? Don't mistake what I am saying, being prepared is wise, but if shopping for all the goodies fills time that could be otherwise spent investing in your relationships, growing spiritually, or obeying God's call for your life, than some serious reflection and changes should occur.

Since our culture teaches women are entitled to have these monumental days, our wedding days and delivery days revolve around our desires, wants, and needs, making us believe they really are all about us. These self-indulgent and self- satisfying beliefs we are influenced by over the years make it difficult to keep our hearts and minds focused on what is truly important in life.

As a Christians, we need to be wary of being self-indulgent. Of course we are going to be drawn to believe we deserve attention and should never experience unnecessary pain. It is self-satisfying and glorifying to feel important and be the center of attention. It is one of the greatest temptations we face.

What we need to realize is that nothing in this life is all about us. Not our wedding days, not our births, nothing. It's all about Jesus.

God brings forth life from us. He has blessed our wombs and chosen us to be the earthly parents of these babies. What a gift and privilege we have. God has promoted us to parenthood. We need to recognize that in all our preparations for delivery, the journey is just beginning. Parenting and having children is not about us; it's about the Lord, about learning how to have a relationship of dependence on Christ, and about allowing Him to help us grow. Our lives are not all about us. God wants a relationship with us, but He didn't save us just for our benefit. He wants us to be an active member of the Body of Christ, functioning as a team. We are to be living on purpose to share Christ, shining our lights for Jesus in all circumstances.

Our childbirths are about Jesus, what He is doing through us, and whom He is choosing to bless us with. If we focus on ourselves, our pain, or our circumstances, it is difficult to focus on the Lord. "When we decide to be our own center, our own king, everything falls apart: physically, socially, spiritually, and psychologically."[4]

Recognizing our lives, our marriages, and our births are not all about us helps us put our focus back where it should be, on Jesus. Then we can begin to fulfill one of our purposes, which is to glorify Him with our lives, in our trials, and in our experiences and relationships.

So if birth isn't all about us, how does one prepare for birth?

How can we allow our childbirths to reflect that they aren't all about us, but rather about Jesus and what He is doing in our lives?

How can we glorify God in our births? How can we praise Him? There are so many different ways. The fantastic thing is that life itself brings glory to God. We can stand in awe of Him and His creation, but there are many different ways to glorify Him and each is unique to each woman's faith.

How can we dedicate it to Him, as our love offering? We need not make offerings or sacrifices, but like any relationship, when someone gives you a gift, you want to thank him. How can we thank God for the blessing He is giving us in a child?

Our Biblical Birthing Heritage

First let's try to have a biblical perspective on birth. How did our biblical ancestors and mentors give birth? And what was the eternal blessing that came from their births? Let's glean from the wisdom in the Word of God on this topic of childbirth.

We have already established that God designed the woman with a special feature, the womb, which really only serves one purpose—to nurture and grow babies. However, women have never been allowed the privilege by God to control when their babies are born. Even today, women have not evolved, as some would like to call it, to have the control to be able to tell their bodies to give birth. If it were up mothers, we would never hear of overdue babies. No, the reality is God births babies.

God declares it is He who births all of creation just as it is He who creates it. "Do you know when the wild goats give birth? Have you watched as deer are born in the wild? Do you know how many months they carry their young? Are you aware of the time of their delivery? They crouch down to give birth to their young and deliver their offspring. Their young grow up in the open fields, then leave home and never return," (Job 39:1-4, NLT).

"Adam made love to his wife Eve, and she became pregnant and gave birth to Cain. She said, 'With the help of the LORD I have brought forth a man,'" (Genesis 4:1, NIV). It was the day God had chosen and ordained to bring a man into this world.

God has created you with this gift, the gift to be a vessel to be used by the Lord, a woman to bring forth another life that has its own purpose and calling. God blesses us with the gift of being able to experience a special bond with Him men cannot. There are other bonds gifted to men. Birth is our blessing from the Lord. Birth is a sacred act of worship. When you offer your body to Christ to carry and nurture another—your child—He gives you the greatest gift, a bond with your child men can't really understand . . . in the same way. As a woman, having a baby is a selfless act, but it is also an eternal blessing. Children are our only eternal inheritance. We cannot take anything in this world with us to heaven, but Lord willing, we will see our children one day there too.

Most of today's culture views children as a burden, not a blessing. A largely increasing number of women believe pregnancy and the event of birth to be a burden or illness to be avoided.

"Behold, children are a heritage from the Lord, the fruit of the womb a reward. Like arrows in the hand of a warrior are the children of one's youth. Blessed is the man who fills his quiver with them!" Psalm 127:3-5

The reality is we are all, to a certain degree, byproducts of our environments. Unless we have been transformed by the renewing of our minds through the power of God's Word, giving us the gift of discernment to see what is not biblical or extra-biblical thinking, unless we have witnessed it in our own lives, we will act in alignment with a slowly cooked frog in a pot of boiling water. We don't even realize the lies we've believed. We don't even see how those lies have infected and clouded our worldviews, and thus our perspectives on the blessings of children and the process of childbirth.

So as we listen to the birthing stories of women friends who in their wisdom may not offer very encouraging or empowering advice, be careful to guard your mind and heart from fearing the birthing process.

"Do not conform to the pattern of this world, but be transformed by the renewing of your mind. Then you will be able to test and approve what God's will is—his good, pleasing and perfect will." Romans 12:2

Let me encourage you that God has a great plan for you. He will be there with you every step of the way. Acknowledge His presence. Give Him the control by allowing Him to be your strength.

After twelve years of birthing babies naturally, all between 7lbs., 12 oz. and 9 lbs., 9.5 oz. and progressed labor ranging from one to nineteen hours—I can testify that women are blessed and privileged to have the opportunity to birth babies. It can be painful, but it is a beautiful pain. God can and wants to be our strength. It isn't always the same pain for every woman, but we need to trust that God knows our pain and He promises to give us what we need to persevere if we ask. He is always present, but He wants us to invite Him, to ask Him to help us as we "bring forth man."

Birth is an avenue in which God can extend His mercy and compassion toward us.

Childbirth can be an intimate experience in which you can personally witness God's healing strength and power. When you experience His healing in such a merciful and compassionate way, your faith grows and you become more loyal and trusting in His grace. You can feel His mercy on your body and the fullness of God's blessing in gifting you with a child, as well as the spiritual growth that comes from relying on Him for strength in a time of intense weakness. As a bonus, you have the added benefit of creating an everlasting memory of your experience with the Lord that will forever change your relationship with Him and the way you approach life.

Our faith that God designed our bodies well to birth babies is under attack. But God's design of our bodies to withstand childbirth is much bigger than our bellies! We must fight to preserve the view that natural childbirth is a rewarding and valuable experience both in our minds and those of younger generations.

Do we dare allow our culture's fears of the birthing experience cloud our vision and create a fearful heart within us, or do we choose to study the Word of God, listen to our bodies, and pursue birth in faith, hope, and trust?

If we don't view life as a sacred gift, then we won't want children simply because we'll focus on the sacrifices (our bodies, sleep, and money) we would have to make based on selfish and worldly perspectives. When birth is under attack, life is under attack. It is like any slippery slope, and we the church need to keep our armor heavily outfitted in this battle so we can "extinguish all the flaming arrows of the evil one," (Eph. 6:16, NIV).

We need to reclaim childbirth in the name of Christ, so we can more easily reclaim sanctity of life in His name. We need to be saturated in His Word so our minds are transformed to be like His . . . viewing children, pregnancy, birth, and motherhood all as blessings, not sacrifices or burdens. If we believe what His Word says is true—that He has created each person uniquely in his mother's womb (Psalm 139), and He has ordained the days of his life from before he was born (Jer. 29)—then we must believe God has blessed you by choosing you to be your child's mother. God designed you to be able to give birth. Claim that truth. If you truly believe God is the creator of life, then rest in peace knowing He is in control of knitting your baby together to be what He sees as His masterpiece. He created your body a beautiful masterpiece designed to do the job of childbirth.

Take a moment and open your Bibles to read Psalm 139:13-16.

God designed you to love deeply, to lean on Him, to need Him, and to have babies. Our souls are designed to yearn for Him to know our deepest thoughts, to judge any grievous way in us and lead us to eternal life with Him. Take joy; you were created by God, designed well to birth children, and to nurture and mother them.

"Yet the Lord longs to be gracious to you; he rises to show you compassion. For the Lord is a God of Justice. Blessed are all who wait for him," (Isaiah 30:18, NIV). The Lord longs to be gracious to you, to show you mercy and grace . . . He longs to be intimate with you. He has provided you with an opportunity to grow in Him. Embrace this opportunity, dear sister, so He may do a preparing work in your heart for motherhood.

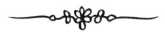

Let's pray

Lord, we come to You fully surrendered and desiring to live all of our lives on purpose. We desire for Your will and plan for our childbirths and the blessings to come to unfold in our lives as women who strive to know You, experience your mercies and love deeply. Please use us to bring Your love and the understanding of Your Word on this topic to more women in the church so all our minds can be unified and come back to Your will to be transformed by Your works. Thank You that there is a big picture, Lord, that these lives we are living are not all about us. Thank You for giving us the opportunity to work on Your team, to be blessed by Your body, and to be filled up to pour out again. Keep our eyes on You. Let us not forget how You love us and so desire to meet us in this intimate experience, which You have designed us for. May every woman who reads on be blessed, and may she feel empowered to seek You and let You be the focus in her birth and in how she shares and encourages other women. Thank You for the eternal focus You have blessed us to gaze upon—that birth is infinitely bigger than our bellies, Lord. Amen.

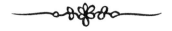

Preparing Your Heart, Soul, Mind, and Body for Birth

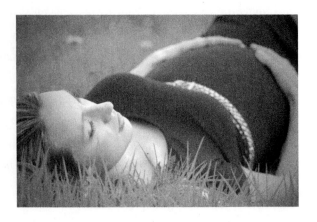

Childbirth is the one time in a woman's life when—without a doubt—she will be challenged in her heart, soul, body, and mind, all at the same time.

> *"You must love the LORD your God with all your heart, all your soul, all your strength, and all your mind."*
> **Luke 10:27 (NLT)**

I have a good friend who runs marathons with her husband. They run and train for months so their bodies are physically capable for the race. Childbirth is like a marathon. It takes purposeful preparation. If you don't prepare emotionally, physically, and mentally for this race, you will get weary and may lose hope and turn to interventions or alternatives that are rarely ideal. But if you focus on the Lord with all your heart and soul, you will find the spiritual endurance to stay the course. What a beautiful but hard concept right? What does that look like, you might ask?

When we seek God and find Him, we receive spiritual gifts such as peace, patience, and self-control. These gifts from the Lord come from trusting and surrendering to Him. Peace alone is a strength that impacts the heart, soul, mind, and body and can only be given to us by God. In times of stress, God can give the body physical peace and calm the nerves. He can bring a peace of mind. He can ease an anxious soul. Jesus can comfort and fill up a broken heart creating a peace that comes from restoration. God can even bring a peace to a soul in the form of confidence. This confidence comes from surrendering everything to Him, not from the situation, the doctors, or our own abilities.

No matter what circumstance arises in labor or birth, patience is a needed attribute in order to endure the race. There are times during labor when a woman grows anxious, waiting for the pain to be over and see the baby, and it is in those moments that patience for God's timing is the most necessary. Patience comes from trusting Jesus, and trust in Jesus comes from knowing Him.

Self-control is another fruit of the Spirit from God that helps us keep our minds focused on Him. In birth, having self-control over the desire to focus on self and indulge ones emotions through screaming and tensing up is crucial to experiencing His presence. It takes controlled effort of the mind and soul to make it through childbirth. You must focus on Jesus and lean on Him to stay the course until the end.

> *"Peace I leave with you; my peace I give to you. I do not give to you as the world gives. Do not let your hearts be troubled and do not be afraid."*
> *John 14:27, NIV*

So how does one receive these gifts of peace, patience, and self-control from God?

The Holy Spirit who dwells within a person who has surrendered to Christ gives each of these fruits. The more you seek Him, the less you will experience the common stresses and worries typically associated with pregnancy and childbirth in our culture.

Practical Tips on How to Prepare Your Heart for Birth

In preparing your heart, remember to have a true picture of how God views you. Debra Evans writes, "You are redeemed, justified, cleansed, guarded, forgiven, blessed, saved from condemnation, and loved beyond measure. God's unshakeable love, mercy, and grace are the solid source for your self-esteem."[5]

Take time to prepare by reading and meditating on the Word of God, praying to Him about your concerns and praying with others as well. Spend time in worship, singing to the Lord. Find a few songs that minister to your heart and soul while praising and glorifying your Father.

If you have an anxious heart about birth, be honest with yourself. Are there unresolved issues in your life? Do you need to reconcile relationships or set boundaries for your health or your baby's? Use this time during pregnancy to pursue healing in your heart.

Be honest and real with others. It is helpful to verbalize what is going on in your heart. If you have past hurts, you need to get them out and communicate them; it is part of a healthy healing process. Talk with your husband, your mother, your friends, your pastor's wife, counselor, and also your midwife. Being forthright with your midwife or labor coach might prove to be beneficial for you in childbirth.

Ultimately, pursuing peace and reconciliation in relationships helps to lighten a burden that can become even more wearisome to carry in birth. As you deal with past hurts or relationships that are currently causing you pain, seek God. Lean on Him and He will provide you the strength and courage you need to pursue peace in a way that glorifies Him.

If you cannot accomplish reconciliation in a relationship, then release it to the Lord. Do what is right before the Lord, and receive His healing touch in your life. Ultimately, we each have our own unique circumstances and if we take them to the Lord in prayer and seek wisdom from His Word, and then pursue to obey His Word, that is all we can do.

You will be blessed more than you know during your birth if you truly pursue peace in your relationships, especially with God.

God loves you deeply and wants so badly to be close to you, His precious daughter. He doesn't like walls in His relationships with any of His daughters. Reflect on your relationship with the Lord. Is there anything you need to repent of and humble yourself before Him to receive His forgiveness and love? Healing of our whole heart can only happen through the power that comes in forgiveness—forgiving others and receiving forgiveness. Jesus paid the price for our forgiveness, and it is free. There is nothing we can do for it. We just have to receive it.

Let your heart be strong, undivided, and undistracted in birth. A light heart will help make a great birth. When your heart is light, you have more room for joy and love; you will not be distracted by all those thoughts that can weigh down your heart.

Preparing Your Mind

Preparing your mind for childbirth is critical to developing your confidence in the ability to give birth to your baby. Our minds are 100% connected to our bodies. Our minds are the control center for what our bodies actually do. So if our minds are distracted in birth, our bodies will struggle. By distracted I mean anxious, thinking about fears, or thinking about relationship problems, thinking about other people's horror stories. Anything could potentially be a distraction.

The Bible warns us to take our thoughts captive. If we do not, we will easily tempted to be indoctrinated by our culture, to be tempted toward fear. Throughout the birthing experience, mental strength is key. You have to have mental strength to prevent yourself from being tempted by fear when you are in excruciating pain. You need mental strength in order to focus on the Lord and His promises, to worship Him, and to pray to Him throughout your birth. The only way to prepare for this mental strength is to exercise the muscle of self-control. As mentioned before, self-control is a fruit of the Spirit that is an asset in an experience such as childbirth. It helps us to reject activities or self-indulgences we know are not good, approved by, or pleasing to God.

What are some examples of how practicing self-control can help equip one for childbirth?

Women can keep their minds focused during labor by reciting Scripture and singing praises. But, to be able to do so you need to memorize the verses and know the song lyrics or practice them well enough they become ingrained in your mind and heart. The key is in your mental memory muscle. It takes discipline to practice these spiritual exercises.

The more you meditate on the word of God, His promises, and His precepts, the more confident you become in Him as the caring Father, the Comforter, and the Deliverer. Your faith is strengthened because you get to know Him by studying His Word.

Spending time studying childbirth, the process, what to expect, and how God designed your body to withstand it, gives you a renewed confidence in God. Knowing why He allows us to experience pain and the blessing in it can give you a mental conviction to let it play out naturally. This knowledge can inspire you to engage in and embrace childbirth. If you can dream and envision the refining process a woman goes through during childbirth and how God designed this experience to better prepare us for motherhood, then you can better embrace the process and reap the benefits.

In every one of my births I came to a place, like every woman does, where I thought, "I can't do this." I had to make a conscious choice to not give into the fear, but to use my mental strength and focus on what I knew I was created to do. Sometimes it takes having that right person in the room to remind you that you can do it, but if you do not have that conviction and belief firmly in your mind, you will most likely give in to the circumstances and the pain of the moment.

Strengthening your mind in these intense moments is essential and possible by keeping our minds in the Word and recalling the truths we know about our Lord and what He has done in the lives of those we know. I recalled the story my great-grandmother told me as a child. Grandma

Vi was born in 1912, got married young, and had her first baby shortly thereafter. She had a hard labor from what she recalled. I remember her describing the doctor coming out of her room to ask my great-grandpa Al if he wanted his wife or his baby (my grandpa Henry) to live. My great-grandpa wasn't too keen on that idea so he literally passed out, according to Gram. The doctor had concluded the baby was stuck. Rightfully so, as Gramma Vi was a tiny lady, only five feet two inches tall and skinny as a pole. Back in the 1930s in the farmlands, the doctor would just break a woman's pelvis and rip the baby out, according to Gram. No medication was given; he just broke her pelvis with a hammer. Well, thankfully my stubborn old gram lived and so did her nine-pound baby boy. Shockingly, she went on to repeat this horror story just two years later when she gave birth to another big boy.

I remembered this story as I was in labor, not from a place of fear, but from a place of great confidence, that if God brought Gram through that, then He would help me birth this baby. Up until the last forty years or so, women had been birthing babies naturally for thousands of years. If they could do it, we should have confidence we can too. We need to have a tough mind. A mind so immersed in the Word of God, it comes with us wherever we go, whenever we go.

We need to trust what we know is true about God and strive to honor and respect Him for who we know Him to be, even in birth. He says, "Don't be afraid, for I am with you. Don't be discouraged, for I am your God. I will strengthen you and help you. I will hold you up with my victorious right hand," (Isaiah 41:10, NLT). If we believe His Word is true, His Word endures forever, why do we fear? Why do we let fear prevent us from feeling His presence? This concept alone could be easily meditated on for nine months as a woman prepares for childbirth.

Preparing our minds for this task requires us to be hungry for truth, knowledge, and understanding, which, in turn, should inspire and motivate us to practice mental strength in childbirth. We need to guard our minds from hearing only horror stories. We need to seek out stories

that can create vision and encouragement for us as women of God . . .
encouragement to seek Him out and let Him redeem our births.

Personal Evaluation #1

On the scale of 1-5 how would you rate the following?

How much do you fear childbirth?   1 2 3 4 5

Your mental confidence in the Lord   1 2 3 4 5

Confidence that you can do this (birth)   1 2 3 4 5

How would you rate yourself on Scripture   1 2 3 4 5
memorization?

After having rated yourself, where do you see the most
opportunity for improvement?

The Lord wants you to lean on His understanding, not your own. Your best weapon in fighting low self-esteem is to be in the Word and memorize Scripture. It is our weapon against the lies Satan tries to whisper to us. "You shall therefore lay up these words of mine in your heart and in your soul," (Duet. 11:18). The Word of God will not be written on our hearts without effort. We have to be intentional about reading the Word and meditating on it as to have it written on our hearts . . . memorized. Then God's Word will permeate into every area of our lives.

Take some time to pray and ask the Lord to help you create an action plan as to how you are going to pursue knowing Him and His word more so you may experience the freedom that comes by having confidence in Him.

Preparing Your Body

As you know, your body is a holy temple. Even though we may know this truth, there isn't a more important season to revisit this truth and evaluate our personal lifestyles. Honoring God with our bodies includes a variety of responsibilities from taking care of our minds, hearts, and souls, to making choices that impact our physical bodies. Making wise decisions in the food we consume, having self-discipline in the area of physical exercise, and choosing to abstain from activities that may cause foolish bodily harm are examples of such decisions.

> *"Do you not know that your body is a temple of the Holy Spirit, who is in you, whom you have received from God? You are not your own; you were bought at a price. Therefore honor God with your body."*
> 1 Cor. 6:19-20, NIV

God created you to provide all your baby needs. In this season of pregnancy, nourishing and protecting your baby is a physical act of worship to our Lord. You are providing a safe haven for the unborn, which is a good work!

We have a common struggle to be self-indulgent. "Honey, can you go get me some ice cream . . . oh, and maybe a taco too?" Let's be honest; we have all been there at least once. We have all experienced those cravings that seem so strong you feel you might not survive unless you indulge yourself. It is easy to make excuses for not doing what we know we should in the area of taking care of our bodies, isn't it? Our culture tempts us to relax in our self-discipline, "Go ahead and have seconds . . . after all you are eating for two." We hear all kinds of excuses from others; exit strategies in taking responsibility. These excuses replay in our minds so frequently we use them to justify many of our actions or lack thereof.

One thing I have learned over the years is that pregnancy and childbirth can take a toll on your body IF you don't take care of yourself. I began having children when I was young and full of energy. In my youth, though I knew I wasn't immortal, my actions or lack thereof in regard to taking care of myself (working out regularly) reflected an attitude of not needing too. I fought those mommy guilt trips created by believing the lies that I wasn't as good of a mom if I wasn't with my child all of the time. Believing those lies led me to sacrifice doctor appointments and exercise.

In the past twelve years of carrying, birthing, and nursing babies I have learned in order to be able to do it well, mama needs to take care of herself first. It is just like the attendants on the airplane teach, "In case of an emergency, mothers of young children need to first apply their oxygen mask, then your child's." The care given and available to a child is only as good as the caregiver can offer. When we are not healthy, we cannot give what we do not have. The same goes for our mental and spiritual health. As mothers, need to take our health seriously.

One mental image that has truly helped me to put my childbearing years in perspective is the image of a race. You cannot participate in a triathlon and expect to do well without having trained or prepared. No, runners train and prepare their minds, their teams and their bodies for the race months before they ever compete. While childbirth is not a competition with anyone . . . it is like a race that will have wear and tear on your body if you do not take care of yourself.

When we take special care of our bodies, we will be rewarded tenfold in childbirth, our recovery, and with the strength to bear more children (if the Lord chooses to bless us in this way).

Preparing our bodies for this season of childbearing is more than just exercising and eating healthy. It also includes healthy sleep habits and lifestyle choices. Life style choices such as standard of living and choice of occupation have huge impacts on the state of our bodies. Financial irresponsibility can cause enormous amounts of stress on women. Stress and pregnancy are not friends. It would be wise to evaluate all areas of one's lifestyle in anticipation of the new blessing and season of life one is entering.

In regard to preparing our lifestyle and body for childbirth, the reality is it takes time and effort. You have to commit yourself to do it. If you are a mother of even one child, you will find taking care of your physical condition gets harder and harder. As mothers, we willingly sacrifice for our children. We believe the lie that if we are gone from our children for even an hour a day to exercise we are being bad moms. We allow ourselves to believe lies that give us guilt. As mothers, we need to think bigger. We need to think ten to twenty years down the road. We need to think about what taking care of our bodies will afford us with our children. We will be more active as parents, we will have better health in general, and Lord willing, we will have longer lives because of it. We need to see that by taking care of our bodies, we are taking care of our children. Involving our children as much as possible in our exercise and daily habits will reap long-lasting benefits for them as they develop their own healthy lifestyle. We need to model this truth that we believe, that God has given each one of us a temple of the Holy Spirit, and that by taking care of our bodies we will be equipped to serve God more fully in our callings in life.

We need to teach a balanced biblical view of this. Taking care of our bodies should never become an obsession that becomes an excuse for not having enough time to nourish our minds, hearts, and souls.

Personal Evaluation #2

On a scale of 1-5 how would you rate the following?

Physical exercise/ healthy activity	1 2 3 4 5
Occupation/ Lifestyle activities	1 2 3 4 5
Sleep habits	1 2 3 4 5
Eating habits	1 2 3 4 5
Stress level	1 2 3 4 5

After having evaluated your physical lifestyle, what areas do you see need most improvement?

Pray about and write down a realistic action plan for creating change:

On a scale of 1-5, what is your level of commitment to change?

If your commitment level is below a four, revaluate your action plan until it is one you can commit to and will succeed at. Choose today to keep your word to yourself in regard to what you commit yourself too. My husband Isaac (http://choosegrowth.com) has taught me this concept: before we can keep our word to others, we need to have developed a habit of keeping our word to ourselves. When you put your mind to something you know glorifies the Lord and He has called you to it, practice having integrity to yourself.

Preparing Your Body for Water Birth

I am a HUGE advocate of utilizing water in pregnancy and birth. I have found that going to the local pool to do exercises while I am pregnant helps with my flexibility, plus it helps being in a zero gravity environment when you are VERY pregnant (i.e. heavier). One can also relax in her own tub at home as well. This provides a great environment for doing squats, pelvic rocks, and other birthing exercises when pregnancy is nearing the delivery date and one is tired and feeling less able to get up and down off the floor or handle doing tons of exercises. There were many times during summer pregnancies when the only thing that helped my body to feel less physical stress was going swimming or soaking in a tub.

Birthing in the pool has many benefits as well. Labor is a workout and often women can find themselves having very quick temperature changes. I have noticed a dramatic difference in my temperature during water birth compared to non-water births. For me, when I am hot from the work out of laboring, the water is cooling. It has always been an opinion of mine that while laboring in the water, one's skin becomes more flexible and elastic. When you spend any amount of time washing dishes, your hands get all pruned up, right? This benefits one's perineum in birth, resulting in less tearing and trauma to that intimate area.

Throughout this book you will read many of my birth testimonies, which include what I experienced in the water. I have had three underwater births and labored in the water for five of my births. If I were to compare the experiences, I would hands down advocate water birth. It is a natural form of pain relief. When a woman has back labor, stepping into a pool of water can offer relief and often help to progress labor by moving the baby. Every time I would stand up for monitoring during my first birth, all I wanted and craved was floating back in the water, simply so I could have relief in my back. The zero gravity environment helped my baby to float up and turn.

A Special Note on Waterbirth

I think that we Christians have a chronic problem with labeling and judging things as "new age" or "hippy" and throwing the baby out with the bath water when those who are secular or of other religious beliefs promote a certain method. As I clearly warn, we do need to be careful about this. We need to be wise, and not participate in activities or exercising that go against the Word of God. But water birth does not do this. It is simply a method. A means to an end that can make the experience less painful and faster. Anything that enables us to have our focus more on the Lord and less on our pain is worthy of consideration.

Women from all over the world birth in water and have for centuries. I am bringing this up for a few reasons: 1) I am an older sister in the Lord who wants you to have a wonderful birth experience and I am simply sharing one method that has helped me numerous times to physically deal with the pain in childbirth. 2) I think that we Christians have a chronic problem with labeling things as "new age" or "hippy" and throwing the baby out with the bath water when those who are secular or of other religious beliefs promote a certain method. As I clearly warn, we do need to be careful about this. We need to be wise, and not participate in activities or exercising that go against the Word of God. But water birth does not do this. It is simply a method. A means to an end that can make the experience less painful and faster. Anything that enables us to have our focus more on the Lord and less on our pain is worthy of consideration.*

---

*   For more information on the benefits of water birth please visit
    http://redeemingchildbirth.com.

Preparing Your Soul for Childbirth

Preparing your soul is a journey of coming to a place of inviting God, through surrender, to redeem your childbirth. A journey of healing your mind from the lies taught to us by our western culture. A journey of transforming our hearts to embrace childbirth for all God made it to be. This is your journey, one that will change your life, not just during childbirth, but forever. When you ask the older generations what made them so tough, they tell stories of the hardships they lived through and how those experiences made them strong. Childbirth is intended to be one of those experiences for women. It is intended to be an experience you look back on, not with bad memories or regrets, but as one you want to share because you experienced God in such a personally strengthening way.

Preparing your soul for childbirth is intentionally getting every fiber of your being ready for this life-changing experience. As women seeking to be fully surrendered to God and to glorify Him in our births, we need to surrender all of our being to Him while we are pregnant and preparing for birth and motherhood. We need to allow God to forgive us, to teach us, to refine us, and to make us grow in His wisdom. We need to pursue a deep relationship with Him through transparent and honest communication through prayer. God has a unique and special plan for each of our spiritual journeys with Him, but He desires for us all to pursue Him and know Him. He loves you so much and has so many spiritual blessings He wants to give you. All you need to do is seek Him sincerely.

God desires for us to be in a personal relationship where we trust Him to provide for all our needs, even in childbirth. When we focus on loving Him with all our heart, soul, mind, strength, and through the actions of loving others (our babies within us and those serving us), the Lord has begun redeeming our childbirths. Jesus is the one who can redeem our childbirths, not us. He can bring restoration and is the one who delivers the babies, and in that He also delivers us from pain. Our pain is over once we give birth. However, just as we have personal responsibility in our relationship with Christ and seeking Him (1 Chron. 28:9, Ps.119:2, Prov. 8:17, Prov. 28:5, Matt. 6:33, 7:7), we also have personal responsibility to pursue the truth about childbirth from a biblical perspective. As followers of Christ, we need to do our part in asking God to redeem our childbirths, allowing Him to feed us the spiritual food we need to grow and mature through His Word. We need to actively surrender and submit our births, our plans, our expectations, our fears, our pain, all of it, to Jesus so He can redeem it and use this experience to bring us through this sanctifying experience.

In Hebrews 11, the infamous chapter of honoring those who by faith believed in or acted in obedience to God, we find a truth about our personal responsibility in seeking Him. Through faith in Jesus and what He did, these faithful men and women surrendered to Him, so He could do a work in them and through them. "And without faith it is impossible to please God, because anyone who comes to him must believe he exists and that he rewards those who earnestly seek him," (11:6, NIV). The forefathers had the strength of faith that is not just honorable and righteous, but also attainable. We are to look to these saints' examples, learn from their mistakes, and pursue living in righteousness, glorifying God by our obedience just as they did.

Just as many Christians yearn to hear their Father in heaven say, "Well done good and faithful servant" (Matt. 25:2), we should also envision and hope for our God to say, "By faith you birthed your baby and it was credited to you in righteousness." We should seek to please our Father in heaven in all we do, every season, every experience, including childbirth.

I was the first of my friends to marry and get pregnant so I had a lot of time on my hands being a new stay-at-home wife. I had a lot to learn, and didn't really know what I was doing. I was scared, unsure, and lonely, but I had Jesus and my husband. I spent a lot of time crying out to the Lord, reading His Word and asking Him to teach me. Slowly He brought new friendships into my life that set a good example for me of what it meant to be a wife and mother. But I had a lot to learn. Ultimately, the Lord was my teacher. He was really all I had outside of my marriage for such a long time, but because He was a faithful friend, I wanted to involve Him in my birth purposefully. After giving birth to my first daughter Kelsey, I realized what a sweet spiritual journey the Lord had met me on and shared with me and I felt so blessed.

As you prepare your heart and mind to seek God and draw closer to Him, I pray you feel Him meeting you on your journey. Surrender your will and ask for God's will to be done in your life. Seek to be humble so you can truly listen to God and hear what His will is in regard to where and how you should plan to birth your baby. Then stick to it, to please the Lord, not men. Seek to have a biblical perspective on birth and an understanding of this miracle He has created within you. The more you gain knowledge on the topic of birth and the creation of your body and that of your baby, the closer you will feel to God and your baby. But in all, understand the Lord has a unique plan for you, not like anyone else's. That is the beauty in it, He wants to walk with you in your life, through this special journey of becoming a mother and He wants to bless you.

Just as you have a soul, so does your baby.

Sometimes with all the fuss and focus our culture puts on pregnancy and the needs of the expectant mothers, women can forget our unborn babies have souls that need to be nurtured as well. This is not something you will hear your prenatal doctor talking to you about, how to begin to train your baby in spiritual disciplines and introduce your baby to her Savior. Our Maker created your baby with a soul, a heart, a mind, a purpose, and a destiny. Isn't that an amazing thought? God designed your baby for His purposes and the Lord knows your baby (see Psalm 139).

It is well documented in medical journals that your baby has the ability to hear your voice and recognize it during pregnancy and after birth. Most medical professionals encourage mothers to read to their babies to help them develop voice recognition and cognitive skills. I believe strongly that because God has known our thoughts before we were born, clearly our babies have thoughts in the womb, and since they have thoughts in the womb, they most likely have feelings and even fears. For most mothers, this awareness, that our babies have souls and can hear and have feelings, motivates us to begin our mothering far before our babies are born.

Since our motherhood begins much earlier than the day our precious bundle is in our arms, we can communicate with our babies and develop a loving connection. This special bond that is centered on a desire to nurture our child's soul and develop a spiritual relationship with them that is leading to the person of Christ is a bond that only strengthens over the years. The sooner we take on this responsibility and privilege, the sooner our children can be introduced to this spiritual blessing.

Communicating with your baby

1) Pray aloud over your baby.

Close your eyes, wrap your arms around and under your womb, breathe deeply, and focus on feeling your baby move inside you. Then begin to utter your requests to the Lord. Pray for your baby's growth until birth, pray for his/her safety in childbirth, pray for his/her soul to connect with God, and for his/her future. Pray for God to mold you to be equipped to prepare your child for the path He has created for him/her. Some of the most amazing movements I felt in my belly happened when I was praying aloud or worshiping the Lord. It was like the baby was participating with me and we were experiencing a deep spiritual connection.

2) Worship with your baby

Throughout your day, play music you can worship to. Sing praises to the Lord. You are teaching your baby how to connect with God in worship. Many mothers, myself included, can attest to witnessing certain babies responding to music by actively moving in the womb. Worship helps to set the atmosphere wherever you are. It is healthy for both of you to be worshipping with your souls, abiding in and experiencing Christ's presence.

3) Read the Word of God to your baby.

You don't need to go get a baby's first Bible and begin to read to him or her, although you could . . . no harm done! Simply read the Bible aloud when you are reading for your own pleasure and engagement with the Lord. Our children need to see us in communion with God to learn how too. If you develop the habit now of reading the Word to your child and continuing your own study of the Word, it will be an easier habit to continue as you adjust to the season of motherhood.

4) Talk to your baby.

Growth in relationships comes through communication. Communication is something you have to do on purpose. When you speak to your unborn child while you are pregnant, you will become intimately aware of his/her presence and the responsibility and the privilege you have as a mother.

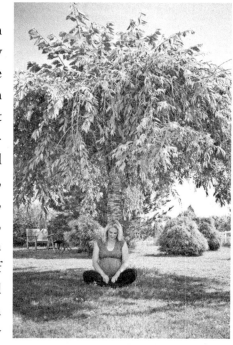

The spiritual connection between the heart, mind, body and soul can be summed up like this: we connect to God through every avenue of who we are at our cores. Our souls are the connection of all of the non-physical parts that make us who we are, such as our emotions, feelings, fears, our knowledge, ideas, vision, and memories, and even our ability to pursue strength of mind. "My soul finds rest in God alone; my salvation comes from him. He alone is my rock and my salvation; he is my fortress, I will never be shaken," (Psalm 62:1-2, NIV). Our souls need rest, and God is the only one who can provide it. Let us find our strength in mind, body, heart, and soul in God alone, allowing Him and inviting Him to be our rock and our salvation.

Preparing your heart, soul, mind, and body for birth and motherhood doesn't stop with this season of life. The habits you are developing today are habits that could potentially sustain you through your lifetime and your children's lives. We as parents set an example for our children of how to take care of ourselves. How we care for our soul by nurturing our spiritual life, our relationships with Christ through devotion, study, service, worship, and prayer will echo into eternity if we proactively and regularly model it for our children.

My secret motivation for taking care of myself in these areas of my life is this: if I want my children to live long healthy lives that are dedicated to serving God wherever He puts them, then I need to be a role model myself. I cannot expect my children to do something that I myself am not willing to do. So as you are preparing yourself, keep the vision of leading your children alive in your mind.

What habits of preparing your heart, soul, mind, and body do you incorporate into your daily life already?

Which habits could you incorporate?

How to Make the Most Out of Your Boot Camp

- Prepare for your birth and motherhood.
- Discover what God's mission is for you in this new season in your life.
- Adopt a vision for embracing birth.
- Deal with fears (Fears can actually have a physiological effect on the progress of birth.)
- Pursue reconciliation in any relationship that you have conflict. (This can also distract and consume a woman's focus and should pursue healing in relationships and healing from past experiences.)
- Prepare your heart, mind, and soul for birth by studying the Word of God and His wisdom.
- Pray and prepare a birth plan and begin a childbirth education class.
- Choose birth attendants with careful wisdom.
- Be flexible. Remember birth doesn't happen on our schedule; allow God to be the one in charge.
- Begin reading books on parenting.
- Pursue finding a mentor whom you trust, respect, and admire. (What does the fruit in her life look like? Do you want your children to grow up to be like hers?)
- Seek out a community of like-minded believers you can raise your children with (if you don't already have community).
- Focus on your marriage and develop good habits of date nights, so that they are sacred traditions kept long after baby is born.
- Check your perspective on children: do you view them as a burden or a blessing?
- Go on a personal preparing retreat/silent retreat by yourself!

Begin purposefully preparing as a married couple for this new blessing soon to be joining your family. I would highly suggest doing some planning and visioning together, like what you do when you are planning a wedding and you go through premarital counseling. Parenthood is a lifelong ministry just as marriage is and it is something worth investing time in to talk and develop a family mission, a vision, and to work out any issues about child training. This is a time for you to prepare. For Isaac and me, it was helpful for us to distinguish the difference between vision and mission. Vision doesn't have to change (like "Leaving a Legacy"), but a mission grows as we do (the action steps, the mission, may look different and change slightly).

You want to be proactive parents, not reactive. Proactive parents have vision and see a few years ahead. Create a regular schedule of dating one another, if you have not already. A new habit is hard to develop, but if you already have the habit it will be much easier to keep it alive and going if you have been practicing it for a while. Another suggestion would be going on a short marriage retreat to get away from all the nesting and focus on the Lord and your marriage.

Personal Preparing Retreat

My friend Lindsay shared a fantastic article at PassionateHomemaking. com on the topic of preparing for motherhood while pregnant. She shares her personal journey of preparing for motherhood and embracing the gift of another child:

> "I have found taking a personal retreat prior to having a new little one to be an invaluable exercise toward preparing my heart for this new stage in my journey of motherhood. Get away, spend time with the Lord, read His word, and pray. Pray for grace. I must acknowledge that this task is certainly beyond my ability. I cannot be a good mother on my own strength. I will stumble and fall . . . time and time again. I need to let go and find grace in His arms."

While on her retreats, she loves to study the Word and prepare spiritually by meditating on the truth that children are a blessing.

"Jesus loved children. He welcomed them. He embraced them, (Matthew 18:2-6; Mark 9:37; Matthew 19:13-15). He promised in His word they are a blessing, a heritage, a reward. They are His generous legacy chosen to be passed down through us. Children are weapons—a tool entrusted into our hands to be prepared to wage war in the enemy's camp. With the influence and power of God's gift of children, no one can stand against us (Psalms 127:3; Deut. 28:4)."

Here are a few suggestions on ways to get the most out of your retreat time:

1) Go alone and try to make it a silent retreat where you are not talking to other people while you are gone, whether it be on the phone or online. Dedicate this time to your relationship with the Lord.

2) Focus on studying the Word of God. Do a Word study.

3) Spend time in prayer and communion with Jesus.

4) Take a good book.
There are so many fantastic books out there. Visit "Nesting in Knowledge" for recommendations on where to get started

5) Spend time asking God to help you to surrender any sin or anxiety in your life. Experience renewal in Him.

6) Worship. Sing praises to the Lord. Think on Him. Meditate on Him. Swim in His presence. Give Him glory!

Take some time and journal a prayer to the Lord, sharing your feelings with Him about childbirth and being a mother. Find someone close to you who will commit to pray for you as you intentionally pursue growing as a woman of God and surrendering your birth and your role as a mother to Him.

Kneeling Before the Porcelain Throne

Sacrifice or Blessing?

Some women have much easier pregnancies than others, but all women experience some level of discomfort both in carrying and delivering a baby. Some consider this a sacrifice and others do not. In light of the fruit, how can it be a sacrifice to bring forth another life? Our culture preaches that pregnancy is an ailment, that it can destroy your body, your sex life, and even your marriage. Today, there are many who primarily look at the cost of having a child versus the blessings a child can bring. We have become so accustomed to avoiding uncomfortable or painful experiences that when a woman hears of others' bad pregnancy-related symptoms, she chooses to forego parenthood. We have to realize God in His goodness blessed us to be fruitful and multiply. He views children as a gift, therefore we should as well.

I do believe when we are living by the Spirit we do not feel receiving a blessing as a sacrifice. In fact we should deeply desire His eternal inheritance found in the gift of a child. However, for some, parenthood and the responsibility of raising a child may require changes in lifestyles and occupations if one was living in the flesh and fulfilling their own desires. The sacrifice to be made for some is a conscious choice to sacrifice ones natural will. Having a child goes against our physical or flesh-selves and this puts us in a spiritual battle as believers.

For some women, God may use their journey in pregnancy to crucify idols of a perfect pregnancy or childbirth. When we lay down our lives and repent and turn from our sin, in sacrificing our will unto the Lord, sometimes we can make the inaccurate assumption that because we surrendered our womb, God is going to give us a perfect pregnancy or birth. But for some of us women, receiving His cross includes accepting nine months of vomiting in exchange for the blessing of bringing forth life.

Bringing a child into the world can bring out the ugly, selfish, sinful heart attitudes in a person sometimes. The realization that life is not all about ME, and that someone else must be cared for first can be scary for some, but for others it can be extremely empowering. Blessed is the woman who has grown in maturity to see that this life will go on long after she will. Blessed is the woman who invests her days building for eternity, for her labor will not be in vain.

The sacrifice can seem more daunting for women who experience hard pregnancies, in which they vomit numerous times per day for most of their pregnancies or are on bed-rest for months with very limited abilities. Through this very difficult and challenging time, it is helpful to note that our God who has the power to stop us from experiencing pain can heal our bodies, and if you are sick, it is because He has allowed it. God does not cause our unfortunate circumstances, but allows them to happen, just as He allowed Lazarus to die, Job to lose his whole family, and the blind man to be healed. There is a greater lesson to be learned, and the lesson is for many more than just Lazarus, Job, or the blind man. The lessons were for Lazarus' two sisters and all who witnessed his death, burial, and Jesus raising him from the dead. The lessons were for Job, his friends, and the community in which he lived. The blind man was healed so all could see the power of the Lord; it was for the advancement of the Kingdom of God.

All of these testimonies we read in Scripture are for our benefit as well. We are to learn from their examples and understand God was brought glory through great pain and suffering. He was brought glory through how Job dealt with loss and suffering. And He was brought glory through the testimonies of deliverance. We do not always know the ways and purposes of the Lord, but we can count on His great love for us and know He is in control. Though I would not compare morning sickness to these examples directly, the point is, what we experience in life, even the bad or uncomfortable, can be for our benefit, and to glorify the Lord. When one focuses on the Lord in all things, our hearts are drawn to find the good in all, to find opportunities for growth.

Through these next two testimonies that are shared, I want to make myself clear: I in no way want to glamorize suffering or illness. I in no way want to make a saint of the mothers who experience morning sickness. The truth I want to express here is very simple: God is good, all the time. In His goodness, He has a plan for each of our lives, and specifically as pregnant mothers if we entrust our lives to Him, He will deliver us. It just may look different for each of us.

A bit ago I mentioned I have struggled with jealousy of friends who seemed not to experience morning sickness. May I say this is a very dangerous trap as expectant mothers and we need not compare. The truth is God has a journey specifically tailored for each one of us. We should rejoice over the works He is doing in our lives and not expect Him to do the same in others' lives.

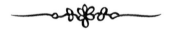

A Story of Deliverance from Morning Sickness

A dear friend of mine shared with me her testimony of God's grace in her life in regards to morning sickness. I was overjoyed when I read it because I felt it was the complete companion to my experience. You see, I feel compelled to share candidly and truthfully about my experience and how hard it was because honestly . . . I felt extremely alone in a community sense. I very rarely met women who experienced such severe morning sickness and were willing to talk about it. In fact, my experience was that I not only felt alone, but I felt like a whimp. Women who never experienced morning sickness, didn't have much encouragement for my particular situation. And when they did genuinely try to encourage me, there was this part of me that couldn't receive it because they had never walked through those countless mornings when you can't get out of bed. They didn't understand the mental challenge it was to be positive about even being pregnant when you feel like you are failing at everything you are doing because your body isn't holding up physically.

I have been there; six times I have been there. Every pregnancy has been completely different, but many might assume since I have six children that I have easy pregnancies. But that is simply not true. In fact my story is one of encouragement for those mothers, who in their despair, need that spiritual encouragement to find the eternal perspective in why I am going through this.

However, my story alone leaves you, the reader, with only being led to think you are doomed to experience morning sickness, which is simply not true. I believe Jesus wants us to live in victory over sickness, but victory will look different for everyone. For some, victory will be in how they praise Him when life is hard; for others, it will be through the testimony of healing.

Ann's testimony of complete healing from morning sickness is truly a testimony of God's grace in her life:

During my first pregnancy, I struggled with morning sickness, like you, for four months. And every day, I fervently prayed for God's help and deliverance.

I know the exact moment God touched me.

One morning at church, an elderly man (a stranger) came up to me and told me, "During worship, the Lord showed me you are pregnant and you have been suffering from morning sickness. The Lord says that you will never have that problem again."

As I heard those words, something inside my heart leaped in faith. I'm serious. I just reached up my arms and instantly said, "I receive it, in Jesus' name!"

Right at that moment, I felt something happen inside me, and from that day (aside from three brief queasy moments), I was completely delivered from morning sickness . . . and not just through that pregnancy, through all seven of my pregnancies. This was God's grace for me. It was a totally undeserved gift and one of the most powerful examples in my life of God's presence and power.

One queasy moment was on a mission outreach in China as our family walked through an open market, with many strange animal smells. The second time was on another mission trip, during a bumpy turbulent flight on a small plane. I honestly think these two queasy moments would have affected anyone, pregnant or not. However, there was one random morning during the last trimester of my seventh pregnancy when I woke up feeling nauseous and horrible. I tried to ignore the feeling, but as I came downstairs, my husband prayed for me and said, "Honey, you don't look so good."

I said, "I don't feel so good. Can you please pray for me?"

Jon laid his hands on me and prayed, specifically rebuking the nausea and sickness and thanking God for all the years of His miraculous healing. Almost instantly, the nausea lifted and I felt completely better. In this instance, I felt sick for about thirty minutes, but never threw up. This third situation, I felt sick for about thirty minutes, but never threw up. This third situation felt like an attack of the enemy, trying to discredit God's testimony of healing my life.

Since God delivered me from morning sickness, over twenty-five years ago, I have rarely felt nauseas for any reason. However, during the time I was reviewing this chapter, I was fishing on a small boat in Alaska with my husband. I became quite seasick for several hours, and although it didn't feel funny at the time, the coincidence seemed so humorous to both my husband and to me. Even as I was sharing my testimony of complete healing from morning sickness, I felt such compassion and mercy for pregnant mothers who suffer with nausea. God is so good, all the time, and He gives us His grace.

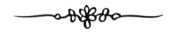

Ann's testimony of God's grace and deliverance from experiencing intense morning sickness shows what the Lord is capable of in all of our lives. He can and will deliver us, in His timing and in His will.

As women of God we need to be hopeful and full of faith that God can and will heal us from all sickness, including morning sickness. We need to submit that desire unto the Lord and willingly receive whatever He has in store for us; whether that be deliverance and healing from sickness entirely or deliverance through it as He provides strength to endure. There is no condemnation whatever outcome you have. If you do not experience healing, it does not mean you have less faith than the woman who has been healed. We are all on our own journeys, which God has planned for us. Whatever our circumstances, we have the opportunity to glorify Him. If you are healed, be thankful and look for ways to encourage other young mothers. If you are experiencing a hard pregnancy, reach out to your sisters to pray for endurance and strength to run this race well, giving Him glory with joy in your heart and praise from your lips.

My dear friend and I have two very different stories. One is of deliverance from morning sickness and one is of deliverance during morning sickness, but both are glorifying to our redeemer Jesus and that is where we have unity. That is where we can rejoice together for what He has done in our lives.

A Story of Deliverance During Morning Sickness

As I shared before, I am all too familiar with how hard morning sickness can be. I have experienced it at different levels during every one of my pregnancies. And I have been right there, questioning, "Why me?" Crying out to God, desperate for Him to provide some reason for why I was so sick. I remember thinking I was through, done, finished. In those moments of literal emptiness, after having purged it all, when all that is left in you is dry heaving you feel you could never do this again, I had conversations with God where I cried out to Him yelling, "Why, after I offered my body to be a nurturing vessel to bring forth life—why would You allow me to be sick again? Why do I have to suffer? Why is it so hard for me to be pregnant? Why can't I just have an easy pregnancy like everyone else I know?" Then I sinned against God, giving Him ultimatums. I told God, "If you don't heal me, I am through. I am not having any more children." Have you been there?

Then in God's goodness, He provided me His wisdom to see the answers to my questions. As I laid there on my knees curled up on the floor crying, after my five-year-old daughter had just been rubbing my back and holding my hair up as I spewed my fluids in the porcelain throne, I saw a glimpse of what He was really allowing. It was beautiful. He was allowing my heart to be humbled. And He was allowing my family to love me through pain and sickness.

We can rest in confidence that if God has allowed any of us to experience suffering of any kind . . . He will not leave us to go through it alone. He has a huge desire to meet all of us in our sufferings, even in our morning sickness. We need to ask ourselves, what is God teaching me right now? Or even being open to realizing a bigger picture . . . maybe your frailty in being sick and needing others is more a lesson about allowing others into your life to serve you. Times such as these are very refining for those being served and enriching on families and marriages, and could be for friendships and the church as well. We all need each other. I personally have always had a hard time receiving help from others. In the first few years of my young adult years, I poured myself out into service, but was reluctant to accept help myself; that was very humbling, and it didn't feel right to me. Over the years though, as we have had the opportunity to serve others in their hard times, I have learned what a blessing it is to be able to serve, to provide what others really truly need. It took many years, but by the time I had my fifth baby I had realized this was one of the ways God was using me in the church, to provide an outlet for others to enrich their experience by serving me within the context of the church family. It was a blessing both to my family and to those in the church who could serve.

For women who have morning sickness, their labor of love begins long before birth. If we allow it to, it can equip us with tools for a lifetime of motherhood. As mothers, our labors may not always look the same, but servant motherhood is a labor of love. If we don't allow God to refine us through the natural experiences He has designed for us to encounter to fully prepare us for motherhood, then we won't reap the benefits. We need to engage the circumstances and experiences God allows us to encounter. We need to understand these trials can make us stronger if we let them, but not if we seek to avoid or ignore them.

The statistic for women who experience morning sickness varies among sources, but averages around 50%. Like most women, every one of my pregnancies varied on the amount of time I experienced being sick. My first baby was very eye opening for me. I struggled with depression largely because I was the first of my friends to get married and then to become pregnant. I had so many dreams and hopes that because I was so sick, I could no longer pursue. I was a newlywed attempting to finish my degree, when I found out I was pregnant with our first baby. I found out because of my "flu like symptoms." After vomiting four to nine times a day for over a week, I went and got a pregnancy test and was excited that it was positive, but also scared. Was this normal to be so sick? Was there something wrong with my baby?

After my first prenatal appointment, I found out it was a good sign to be sick and it was perfectly normal. Feeling great relief, I continued to vomit all the way up until just after I delivered Kelsey. One last final heave, I guess. Each pregnancy has been different; it is not predictable like doctors like to try to say. It has not proven itself to be different based on the sex of the baby, or my diet. I just get sick. I know some women who never have a day of sickness. While a part of me has experienced jealousy of those blessed women who don't get sick during pregnancy, I know God allowed my family and me to go through what we all went through together for a reason. I now know that it served to refine us, and strengthen our faith and family unit. It wasn't easy to see those blessings in the midst of hugging that porcelain throne, mind you, but there was a purpose.

God was teaching me patience and perseverance as I struggled all day with morning sickness. I had to surrender my schedule, my standards for homemaking, and all other idols to Him, which was so healthy for me. Though God did not choose to deliver me from morning sickness, as He has others, He did deliver me from other sins (selfishness, etc...) through this experience.

The labor of love began for me when I was vomiting and trying to keep my focus on the positive—having a baby. It made the thought of being sick seem somehow worth it all. The more I focused on that truth and asked God to reveal Himself to me, the more I grew. Every day as I woke up vomiting and went to bed vomiting, day after day, I prayed for my baby, for myself, and for my marriage. Sometimes, that is all I could do. After all, I was already on my knees. For me, that was the physical boot camp God allowed me to experience... being on my knees in front of that old porcelain throne sometimes around sixteen times a day, other days only once or twice. That was what I needed to learn to prepare me for childbirth and motherhood ... to be on my knees crying out to God in prayer, giving it all back to Him, asking Him for strength to endure. Prayer is one of the most powerful ways to communicate with God and is essential in a mother's tool bag.

I want to share something very personal with you that maybe you can relate to. I am a very busy lady and I hate wasting time not doing anything productive. It drives me nuts. I recognize we have only been given a certain amount of days and hours here on earth to do what we were created to do, and I don't want to live with regret. I don't want to waste my life. So knowing this about me, now envision me, day after day, physically drained, lying around, struggling to speak without getting sick. I laugh when I think of all the reasons why this was a good experience for me. The Lord wanted to meet and teach me to stop trying to take control and to trust Him. Those times when I was sick I felt the farthest away from God and yet the closest to Him. I felt the farthest away when I was struggling to understand why, but the closest to Him when I was on my knees desperately praying. The Lord would give me glimpses of hope when I would have a day of no nausea or vomiting here and there.

It was so hard to see the good in something as terrible as vomiting. It is more common today to look at the bad times, the sufferings, the trials, the pain we experience in the "glass half empty" perspective. We don't approach life as a schoolroom with lessons to learn along the way. But as Christians, if we want to glorify the Lord and praise Him in what we perceive as difficult times then we need to look for the good He is doing in our lives as a result of the trials and see the glass as half full. We need to have faith in His plan for us and pray that He wills for us to be filled up.

In those times when I was just so sick that all I could do was lay on the sofa and cuddle my children, I would cry in my heart for them. When they wanted me to talk and answer questions, I struggled. I knew if I did talk it was going to send me to my knees again so all I could do was pray in my mind and cry out to God to help me be what my child needed me to be at that moment . . . and if I couldn't, I prayed for Him to be what my child needed.

This is the experience of laboring through pregnancy, whether it involves bed rest to keep the baby safe in the womb a little longer or vomiting for three to nine months. I found that after having been so sick, my perspective on the sleepless nights and the aches and pains associated with pregnancy changed. I found I no longer chose to give those symptoms power over my thoughts, though they were there, believe me.

This is the vision I want to share with my sweet young friends who struggling with morning sickness—don't let it get the best of you. Choose joy and choose to rely on God. When you are brought to your knees, embrace the road you are on and pray. Let prayer be strengthened in your relationship with the Lord. Keep your focus on the fact you are receiving a gift, and this gift of a child brings another gift—motherhood—that is a labor of love that never ends. Be thankful every day you are sick that you have been given a gift from God in this child. Many women today struggle so much to have children, so be thankful. God is allowing you to be reminded of this gift every day!

Choosing Joy and Being Real

Does being real with your friends and honest about your morning sickness mean you aren't glorifying God? Does it mean you are negative? Of course not, we all need to practice sharing the full truth of who we are, being real. It's ok if you don't feel well in front of your friends; they are your sisters in Christ and they need to know how to pray for and encourage you. This is also an opportunity for them to serve you as well. Choosing joy doesn't mean you hide the truth of what you are experiencing. Not at all. When people asked me how I was feeling, I was completely honest; however I chose to have a smile on my face. Is that fake? No! Because you are choosing to have joy and not let how you feel get the best of you. Keeping a positive attitude and not allowing the morning sickness to get the best of you is part of the refining process some women experience in pregnancy. It is difficult when you are not feeling good, to keep a vision to fight the good fight mentally and emotionally and conquer something that will literally suck the joy from you, but it's so rewarding as you experience the power of your faith in action.

The challenge is to choose to be joyful around your home, with your children and husband. I know this can be a challenge. It is much easier to be joyful with friends you only see every now and again. I would like to encourage you in this because we mothers are God's catalyst for setting atmosphere in our homes. "If Mama ain't happy, ain't nobody happy." In fact, we can purposely shine our lights for Jesus as we look at the glass half full. We should choose to be joyful instead of have a pity party during challenging times because the more we do the more we glorify our Father in heaven. In these circumstances, it takes making the conscious choice to praise Him and be thankful regardless of how we are feeling. When you are on our knees before that porcelain throne . . . allow God to redeem that moment by praying and choosing joy. You may not be able to smile, but ask the Lord for His Holy Spirit to make His countenance shine upon your face. Praise Him for He has made you beautiful and you are with child, a gift beyond compare.

If you have other children and are struggling through morning sickness again, I want to encourage you to focus on setting an atmosphere of worship in your home. We always have worship music playing in our home, regardless of the season or day of the week; it is all we listen to. What we put into our minds, what we listen to, watch, or think about all impact our heart attitudes and core feelings. When I was pregnant, I was especially thankful for the help of the Lord in setting the atmosphere through worship music. On those days when I was in my pajamas at 4:00 pm, struggling to get dinner cooking (because the smell made me nauseated), I was amazed at how much my children were able to get accomplished and how their spirits were not affected negatively though I was feeling so crummy. I believe it was largely because of our focus on Lord at home through the worship music, which set the tone and played throughout our day.

Another great suggestion for those who have children already is to be honest with your children. Make them aware but not fearful of having children and be honest about your struggles. Ask them to pray for you and to help out more around the house. Share with them how excited and thankful you are for the blessing of another baby. As your children watch you sacrifice for the new baby and see that you cannot do as much, they will feel more needed to help out and automatically more connected and loving toward the baby. It is so beautiful, isn't it? I was always afraid I would scare my daughters out of having kids simply from them witnessing how sick I got. What is so amazing to me-- and this is totally by God's grace and not my doing at all—is that they talk about wanting a lot of kids. They honestly see children as a blessing; they believe it because they have witnessed mom willing to make every sacrifice for another life. We value each child so much that a few months of vomiting and bed-rest are worth another's whole life and eternity. One way God can redeem your pregnancy is by the life lessons and heart transformations His Spirit can accomplish in the hearts of our children and others who witness Him working in your suffering. That is not something that can be easily taught, it is caught through living your life as an example to your children. So keep focusing on Him and purposely setting an atmosphere that is centered on praising Him in your home. And don't forget to ask Him to help when it seems really hard to do yourself.

A Letter to a Mom Needing Encouragement

If you are one of those moms struggling with a weak body from excessive vomiting and running to the porcelain throne repeatedly, and you can't even get out of bed to get ready for the day because you are feeling crummy, you are not alone. There are moms who have been where you are. You may feel like you are the only one of your friends who does not have an easy pregnancy and may wonder, "Am I just a wimp?" It isn't an easy road and neither is mothering. This is where your personal labor of love begins. Submit yourself to God, seek Him for strength. He is putting you on your knees, so talk to Him, even if it means lying silently on the floor next to the ol' pot. Your pregnancy is such a short time in comparison to the lifetime of your child.

Keep your focus on God and remember this: nine months of vomiting is a small sacrifice for another person's whole life and eternity.

This truth kept me in perspective. Oftentimes people would be baffled at how I could smile at church while I was racing to the washroom. Honestly, all I know is that was not of me. If it were up to me, if I were choosing an easier life, I probably wouldn't have had six sweet children. The thought of that devastates me. And I wasn't wearing a fake smile either; that is not my nature. I wear my feelings on my sleeve. No, my smiles were genuine because God gave me a vision of what was to come and I would hang onto that as tightly as I could. I meditated on the fact that any amount of vomiting was worth another child's life. God put the joy in my heart, but I chose to protect and not let it get stolen from me by my circumstances. You can choose that too!

Do not lose heart and give up asking in faithful prayer for God to deliver you from morning sickness. If it is in His will for you, He will do it.

Let me pray for you dear sister,

Lord Jesus we thank you for the gift of motherhood and the blessing we have as women to carry our babies in our wombs. We are so thankful for that privilege. Lord, you teach us in your Word we have not because we ask not; and you also teach we will be blessed with whatever we ask in your name if it is within your will. Lord Jesus, if it is in your will for my sister to receive healing from her morning sickness, I pray you would grant her deliverance right now in your name. Help us be women who remember to continually ask for your blessings and to praise you when you answer them, whether the answer is what we so deeply desire or not. Lord, help us to be thankful and to choose joy even when we feel like we can't. Help us to encourage other mothers with edifying words and acts of service when they aren't feeling well. Jesus, let us not forget what you have done for us and of the power in your name, that we may grow in you, whatever journey you have for us. Amen

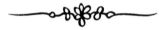

A few things to meditate on

1) Choose to protect the joy the Lord has put in your heart, but be real in the process and allow those God has put in your life to minister to you; let His church be His hands and feet.

2) If you are queasy or vomiting, cry out to Him. If you are already on your knees, use this time to develop a stronger discipline of prayer.

3) Purposely set an atmosphere in your home that reflects the light of our Lord.

4) Keep the faith. Focus on these truths: God loves you and wants you to grow in Him, nine months is a short time to sacrifice for another's whole eternity, life is not all about us and there really is no comparison, keep it all in perspective.

5) It is ok to wrestle with God and cry out to Him. Being a Christian is not all about blind obedience without questioning. Sometimes you need to get into it with God and that is when He can really speak His truth to you.

6) What truths or life perspectives is God trying to teach you? To slow down, to stop and talk with Him, to fully depend on Him, to submit, to be real, to receive service and help in humility, or to believe in Him enough to receive His healing touch?

For a Free PDF Download of Natural Homeopathic, Nutritional, and Herbal Remedies to help with morning sickness visit: redeemingchildbirth.com/

The Unrest that comes with Bed-rest

"I am failing my kids!"

"I can't do this on my own!"

"We barely got any of our school work done in the midst of the midwifery appointments and the morning sickness . . . how am I going to have the energy to make dinner yet too . . . and oh, that laundry has been in the washer for two days now . . . I have to move it over, but the smell might make me puke."

As a home schooling mom who had six babies in twelve years, I have struggled with thoughts like these. Since I have had to be on semi- and full-bed rest for two of my pregnancies due to sickness, I have had those dark days wondering if I was failing my kids. I wondered, if God had called our family to home school, why was I on bed-rest? If God had blessed us with these other children, couldn't I do my job and take care of them the way I had felt called to? I couldn't clean, cook, change diapers, or carry my babies up stairs and put them in their cribs. I couldn't put the toddler on the potty-chair, let alone think of getting any laundry done. I remember one day just breaking down in tears because my eldest daughter's back was hurting her from putting the toddler in and out of the crib and carrying him around for me all the time, constantly handing him to me. I didn't want her to look back on her childhood, remembering me as a sick mom who couldn't take care of her and her brothers and sisters. I didn't want her to feel used or like she had to do the entire grunt work because I couldn't. While many of my friends had family members close by who were able to be a consistent support, we had a very different reality. I struggled with the Lord, wondering why He didn't at least spare me from all the pain and limitations that came with pregnancy if I had been so willing and open to receiving His blessing in another child?

Once our physical needs got extreme enough to humble me, I finally admitted failure in my mind and asked the church for help. Why was it so hard for me to ask for help? And why did I have to admit failure before I could receive help? Why couldn't I simply receive help? Why did I view it as failure? It was pride. I was so used to people judging us for having a large family, I thought that we might get more comments from people if they thought I couldn't take care of them all. I was so tired of people's opinions and didn't want to deal with more voices in my head telling me I was a failure. Just as I was at the lowest I had ever been as a mother and wife, the Lord blessed me by bringing very special older women into my life, to speak life and truth to me.

I was so blessed by these wiser women from our church who came to minister to my family. One dear friend, Sono, shared, "I remember while I was pregnant with the twins, it was difficult taking care of the older children and all of the responsibilities, I had times when I was down and felt the same way . . . but God had a special lesson for each of my children to learn during that season in our family's life." I was so blessed by having an older woman in my life when I needed it most, to speak to me hope, truth, life, and the promise of growth.

Weeks went by after being on bed-rest, and I slowly began to recognize the good that was happening in my family. It took having dear friends like Stephanie come into my home, serving my children every day for weeks, and her blessing me with praises. To have another woman in my home, whom I respected, seeing the good, the bad, and the ugly all day, and still have nothing but kind and nice things to say about my family, helped me gain perspective. She was amazed at how helpful they were and that they enjoyed it. You see, I began to notice the importance in each person being needed within a family. My oldest daughter, who was nine at the time, took over cooking as many meals as was necessary. She cleaned, she changed my fourteen-month-old's diapers, she helped keep the kids busy doing what I asked them to do. She was a huge blessing. My oldest son was six at the time. He too changed his baby brother's diapers and learned how to put him to bed gently, read him books, start our fire in the fireplace by himself, and help take care of the chickens and dog on his own. The younger three were all under four and a half, busy as could be, but so uplifting to me, as they would help do chores and make me things. Everyone rose to the occasion, but still I felt guilty. I felt I was failing them and asking too much of them.

You want to know something ugly? I even dared to question if we were right to have more children. So many people had their opinions on that topic, and everyone seemed so inclined to share it with us too. I am sure while their intentions were good and loving at the core, the reality is their comments felt as judgment and disapproval. I fought those ugly thoughts like, "If I weren't pregnant, I could be taking my kids to that field trip," or "If I weren't pregnant, I would be able to take a meal to that family." And slowly I would come up with as many reasons as time allotted me as to why we hadn't heard God right in accepting another blessing from Him. I was in a battle; my spirit and my mind were under attack.

While these thoughts were racing in my mind, I would make myself sicker. You know that gut feeling you get when you are deliberately about to disobey, or when you were a child and you were about to tell a lie? Every time I would think these negative thoughts, believing what everyone around me wanted me to believe, I would get that gut feeling, like I was in sin for even letting the thought enter my mind. I am so thankful for all the older, wise women I had in my life in that season of trial; they spoke truth to me and helped me to think less selfishly and more biblically. By pointing me to the Word of God, I began to see that we really were in obedience and that God was in control. There was a lesson to be learned in this for me, for my husband, my children, and even those around us who thought they were speaking wisdom but were clearly just experiencing blurred vision.

There we those early moments of feeling I was failing my children, but then as time went on I saw my children thrive as they were expected to do more around the house. We had always believed in giving them responsibility but I was forced out of necessity to allow them to do things that maybe I always just did because I thought they couldn't or I just simply thought I could do it faster. I learned kids thrive when they have a purpose and when they are needed. When we let them be an active part of the team: The Family Team. God was doing something in each of our hearts through this experience.

Another honest introspection is that I have a hard time slowing down. Pregnancy tends to rock my world and slow me down completely. I saw during one of my pregnancies how God slowed me down to help me notice that one of my children needed more sitting time reading quietly with Mommy. It was all I really could do, and within that time, that child began to really enjoy reading and thriving versus struggling. There were so many deeper good things that came out of me being on bed rest, things that might not have happened if I weren't forced to lie still.

My encouragement to you, mom, is that sometimes we don't and can't see the lessons God has in store for our children, our husbands, or even those outside our family. He wants to grow them and prepare them for the future He has in store for them as well. We don't know what that future is, but I rest in knowing the Lord is providing those lessons they will learn from, to make them stronger. I look back now on my time on bed rest, with memories of deep spiritual growth and team growth for all of us.

I wouldn't trade that for anything in the world, not even a normal sickness-free pregnancy. God allowed me to go through what I did, and because I surrendered to it, I was blessed to watch the blessings that occurred within my family and my children's lives because of it.

When I could not be the one training and teaching my children the lessons because I was in the hospital, God did. He taught them and comforted them.

The Bible says, "Train up a child in the way he should go; and when he is old he will not depart from it," (Proverbs 22:6, NIV).

How do you train up a child when you are on bed rest? How do you train up children in today's culture to love the Lord with all their being, so they can withstand temptation, so their faith will endure the hardships of life? We have a promise from the Lord that can bring us hope, that if we train up our children in the way, they will live in the way.

"To train" literally means "to develop or form the habits, thoughts, or behavior of (a child) by discipline and instruction."[6]

To begin with, we need to have grace with ourselves to let go of any pride we may have with regard to being the mother. We should understand that to train a child in the way he should go means we need to know the way we should go. We need to be pursuing truth, continually working on our disciplines of study in the Word and service to our Lord. We need to lead by example. Faith is not just taught; it is caught. If you want your children's hearts to follow after the Lord, wherever He leads them in life, then your heart needs to follow after the Lord. It is so much easier to train your children up in the Lord when there is so much to be thankful for and times are easy and blessed. I find that I had a harder time staying positive and seeing the good to train them up in while I was suffering. In the midst of uncertain trails it is so hard to keep focused on the good. This is our opportunity as parents though, to grow in this ourselves, but also to teach and train by example. As our children watch us suffering and still praising God and thanking Him, they will see true faith.

We need to engage our children and be intentional with walking through life with them beside us. They need to see us handling life's circumstances with grace and hope, praising Jesus in the midst of our troubled times. It is when we allow them to walk through life with us and we intentionally mentor them through discussions, prayer, and study of the Word, that they will be prepared in the way they should go. It is then we can rest in the promise that "when he is old he will not depart from it." Struggling through juggling all the physical feelings, emotional feelings, and spiritual feelings we as women face when we are pregnant allows us a new opportunity to engage our children, to really teach them proactively how good we really believe God is.

We need to praise Him right after we vomit. When you walk out of the bathroom and your kids all have scared looks on their faces, reassure them you are fine and that it is normal and that the baby is fine. Thank the Lord in prayer or put on worship music. Help them view pregnancy as normal because it is normal. Use it as a teaching tool. Engage them, read book on babies, how they are made, and how they are born. Use this as an opportunity to talk to your older children about puberty, sex, intimacy, marriage, and childbirth depending on your child's maturity level. Teach the little ones appropriately.

Lastly, be encouraged that your sufferings are not just for your benefit, or even family benefit, but maybe for the benefit of others, whom you may not have met yet.

> *"Praise be to the God and Father of our Lord Jesus Christ, the Father of compassion and the God of all comfort, who comforts us in all our troubles, so that we can comfort those in any trouble with the comfort we ourselves receive from God. For, just as we share abundantly in the sufferings of Christ, so also our comfort abounds through Christ. If we are distressed, it is for your comfort and salvation; if we are comforted, it is for your comfort, which produces in you patient endurance of the same sufferings we suffer. And our hope for you is firm, because we know that just as you share in our sufferings, so also you share in our comfort."*
>
> *1 Cor. 1:3-7 (NIV)*

I was personally encouraged by older women who have gone before me, in suffering, to share perspective, wisdom, and encouragement. They helped me focus on God and on the good things He was doing through this trial. Now my prayer is my struggles would not be wasted, that they would glorify my King, my God for the good He has done in my life. I pray my testimony has blessed you and encouraged you, and that one day, you would be able to share what you have learned, the testimony of God's hand in your life would encourage other younger women as well, all for the benefit of the Kingdom of God.

A Little Note for Homeschooling Moms

Mandatory bed rest, vomiting, and postpartum hemorrhaging are not what women expect to experience during pregnancy, but when they become a reality it can be a spiritually dark journey for some. Fear of getting behind in school, feeling like a failure as a mom and educator, or even just feeling guilty for not being able to keep up the house or daily routine can all be extremely hard and humbling on an expectant mom. But God wants to embrace you, to lift you up and to teach you about His goodness in new ways that you could never learn about if you had it easy. Look for those lessons. Look for those truths and promises. Look for God in the midst of these hard times.

Allow the body of Christ to minister to you and your family and let your children see what it is supposed to look like. Let the church be God's hands and feet. I know my children were so blessed by all of the women who came and helped in our home while I was on bed rest. They got to see community. God's love and provision in action. No matter what the world says, I know that the Lord did an amazing work in the lives of my children, my husband, and my marriage because I was on bed rest and we were forced to come together even more as a team. I don't regret any of the educational decisions we made during that season. My children grew up and loved serving and they thrived being needed. The education was hands on, service oriented, and focused on the Lord.

We did a lot of praying as a family, more than we ever had before. During this season our children saw firsthand and talked to us about how precious a life is and saw us live out our beliefs, even when it was hard. We talked with them, explained things in depth to them, and spent hours praying with them. And when the Lord granted me the mercy to enjoy the last few months of my pregnancy off bed rest, they saw that as a true blessing, not to be taken for granted. The kids still thank God for healing my back enough that I could walk again. Those lessons cannot be taught by anyone else the same way.

Once your baby is born it is not uncommon to feel overwhelmed by the responsibilities that have been waiting for you as you recover. Give yourself a grace period. Embrace and enjoy your new little one, teach your children how to let the other stuff go, and be flexible and focus on what is most important in life. Let them develop a special bond with their new sibling. Teach them all about taking care of babies, which is so educational. Believe your children are going to be fine—better than fine! They are getting real hands on life experience with a real baby brother or sister. They are getting experience in being selfless while they serve their family. They are learning more about teamwork as they work together to get the simple things in life completed. Praise your children, pray with them, cuddle them, and read to them and you will be doing a great job, so engage your blessings guilt free!

As you lean on Christ to give you strength, glorify and give Him the credit—in front of your kids, know you are doing the work of the Lord. You have sacrificed control for a blessing in this precious life. This is part of why we are at home with our children: to teach them about the reality of life, so they are better prepared and equipped. So equip them; be transparent with your struggles and share what God is teaching you. This can be a time when so much spiritual growth can happen in your family.

Smile, take a deep breath and thank the Lord for this awesome opportunity for stronger family ties. Recognize that though you feel like a failure, God does not see you that way, and neither does anyone else. Don't let the enemy feed your mind with self-pitying and destructive lies. Lean on Him, on His Word and seek Him in prayer. He wants so desperately to empower you. He sent His Spirit to be with us, to guide, comfort, and counsel us. May you receive His unshakeable and uncontainable joy.

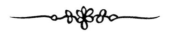

Join me in prayer

Lord, You are the comforter, the counselor, the only one who can bring forth life, the only one who can redeem a bad experience or event and bring forth goodness and truth. May You give peace, joy, and strength to my sisters who are struggling now. Please meet them in their darkest hours; in those hours of feeling like a failure I pray you would speak truth to their hearts through your Word and through your people. I pray you would take these hard times of suffering and pain and use them for your glory. I pray you would transform these times into something that is good and brings truth, light, and growth. May it be a light to all they meet. Help my sisters to have faith that no matter how hard, how difficult, how lonely they feel, You are still with them. May they lean on You and experience growth in their relationship with you through this experience. May You redeem and bring forth something good from their experience. Let not our trials be for nothing, but let us bring you glory as we experience the trials and sufferings of this life.

Thank you for this opportunity to serve you in this way. May we all embrace this season of childbearing gracefully.

Amen

Deceitful Propaganda

As we have mentioned before, redeeming childbirth is something only the Lord can do since He is the only one with the power to redeem anything. However, in order for us as Christians in today's culture to see the need for Jesus to redeem childbirth, to take back something that has been lost to this world, we have a need to recognize truth and turn from worldly perspectives. We need to see the lies our culture has been teaching us with regard to childbirth. We need to recognize self-indulgent trends and choose to stand apart in how we birth. We need to be careful not to compartmentalize birth out of our spiritual lives, but instead glorify Him by how we birth our children. This chapter is focused on revealing some of today's most commonly taught perspectives regarding birth and exposing the truth.

Fears Based on False Teachings

I feel compelled to warn you of false teachings on the topic of child-birth. If you were to go online or to a local bookstore for example and you searched for books on birth, you would find hundreds, all similar in that they describe the stages of labor, how to cope with pain using different methodologies, and what to expect. All of these can prove to be very helpful. I have compiled a list of Christian books on childbirth that I highly recommend that also cover these aspects.

You can print out a free pdf titled "Nesting in Knowledge" with the list at redeemingchildbirth.com/

However, there are deceptions within many literary and educational books on childbirth as well. Deceptions Christians should filter through the Word of God or guard their hearts from entirely. For Christian women who want to invite God into their experience, we need to be careful not to allow the new age beliefs or secular world views taint our perspectives, expectations or preparations for birth. For the deadly philosophies and beliefs about birth today are not the results of human intelligence and inspired thinking, but instead thinking that is unyoked from the true knowledge that comes from the inspired Word of God. We need to practice guarding our minds by actively engaging in the disciplined study of the Word of God.

Be Wary of the Wayward or Lazy Doctor/ Midwife

Guarding our minds from the influence of the world also means we need to be able to filter man's words well, since all things potentially can influence our beliefs. This is extremely critical since our beliefs, those things we believe to hold truth, greatly impact our choices and actions in life. Unfortunately, there is also a need for us to be wise with regard to whom we listen to and take advice from. The truth is that world views greatly impact what we believe. We are so used to just separating our medical care from our faith, but Jesus came to heal and save the lost. He did miraculous healings during his ministry on earth; then went on to tell us we would do even greater miracles. I believe there is a huge need for the medical profession, when someone is in need of it. The advances the medical field has is one main reason our mortality rate is so much lower than it was before hospitalized births. They are able to deal with emergencies such as obstructed labors very quickly and safely.

The medical profession and midwifery schools all have their own unique philosophies and worldviews. Whether they intentionally try or not, their students are somewhat indoctrinated by their education and environment. As Christians, we need to be aware of this so that when we are choosing our professional birth attendants we make wise decisions. Just as we need to filter through the books we read, we should also be wise on who is going to be educating and encouraging us. Finding a health care professional, midwife, and/or doula who has a like-minded worldview about birth and faith can be greatly helpful, especially for first time expectant parents. If you are pursuing a natural birth, it is wise to choose a birth attendant who is an advocate for that. If you choose a doctor who has a record of medicated births or caesareans, you should assume having the natural birth you desire may be discouraged or at least not encouraged like it would be if you had chosen a health care professional that has a record of being a natural birth advocate. If a woman is not very familiar with pregnancy or birth, it is wise to choose someone who will teach you in accordance with your faith, rather than potentially against it. Be wary of the wayward doctor or even wayward midwife.

Another type of doctor I feel compelled to warn you of is the lazy doctor. The lazy doctor is one who chooses the most extreme intervention for the sake of time, money, and convenience. I don't want you to get the impression that I have a negative view of doctors—quite the contrary. When needed, we use them. However, I have personally met a lazy doctor or two. They viewed me more as a number, rather than as an individual. The unfortunate reality is that most of us grow up feeling that way from our doctors and dentists, so we don't see anything wrong with it. But there is something wrong with it. And you do have a choice. There are many good doctors and midwives out there who love what they do and are not self-focused, but genuinely care for their patients.

During my first baby's birth (shared earlier), we experienced a lazy doctor coming in telling us we needed a caesarean. Can you imagine? Yes, Kelsey was good sized for a first born—she was 8.5 pounds—but I have now given birth to six children naturally with three of them well over the nine pound mark he was so concerned about and ready to do a caesarean over. The point is, he had no real reason for suggesting a caesarean, but we used discretion and did what we felt was best for our family. Ultimately, everyone needs to do this. Sometimes there are legitimate reasons for a caesarean, for sure! Unfortunately, sometimes the doctor has a soccer game to get to. Unless there is a real danger to the life of the baby or mother, birth can be done naturally. So just be wary, that's all. Realize you can have a great birth in the hospital; I had four great births in hospitals. You just need to plan to do so.

Do not assume every doctor is wayward or lazy. My intention in writing this section is not to disenchant you toward hospitals or the medical profession, but rather to enlighten you and bring to light facts we are not necessarily all aware of. As Women seeking to have a perspective on pregnancy and birth that glorifies the Lord and rightly places Jesus in the seat of authority over all our decisions, we walk a fine line. On one hand, we need to have a realistic view of medicine and interventions as well as their potential side effects; not relying too heavily on them as to make idols out of them. But we also need to have thankful hearts and respect for the medical advances, the knowledge, and the skills sets the medical profession can offer us in times of emergencies.

The balance we can find comes down to this one basic truth that we can all cling to: seeking Him alone and His wisdom through prayer, study of Scripture and mentoring of like-minded believers; but it is all about Jesus. When we have deep confidence and faith in God's creation of our bodies to carry, nurture, and birth babies without need of such interventions, we are free to make decisions without the bondage of fear.

How do we know if we are making decisions based on the influence of this culture, selfishness, or fear it has created? We need to look deeply at our motives. Why do we need to birth in a hospital? Why do we need to have a home birth? While neither is bad, what is important is the motivation behind why you chose that environment. Whether you are leaning toward choosing to have a hospital birth, a home birth, an epidural, or a natural birth . . . it needs to be for the right reasons. We need to examine our hearts. Are you struggling with making home birth or natural birth an idol? We shan't pursue doing anything good in vain. God humbles the proud. Are you going to doctors or midwives first instead of the Lord, putting them in authority over your decisions, instead of the Lord? Our God is a jealous God. Are you making decision based out of fear? Or do you have legitimate reasons to have fear? We should not make a decision foolishly or arrogantly, but rather wisely. The only way we can truly make a wise decision is to go to our Father.

The Lord wants us to have a deep faith in His design of our bodies to nurture and birth babies. He wants us to lean on Him in all our decision making throughout life, including how, when, and where we have our babies. He wants to help you make a wise decision. Unfortunately, there is no right way for every woman. The only right way is what she feels confidently the Lord has given her peace about. So I encourage you to seek Him, listen to Him, and pursue walking out a strong faith in Him through this journey. He wants to guide you. He wants to show the plans He has for you. When we maintain a healthy biblical perspective of pregnancy and childbirth, we take a real look at our motives and choose to ask God for guidance we can then make confident insightful decisions.

Pregnancy and childbirth alike are not burdens or ailments to be avoided or treated, rather seasons in life meant for growth and blessing. There are many doctors who choose their vocation because of a calling in their lives and they can be a real blessing to you. Doctors do have much knowledge and expertise in dealing with emergencies, so if you have a legitimate high-risk pregnancy, don't be foolish; accept their help and guidance. Their job as doctors is to deal with health issues. Just recognize childbirth in general isn't a health issue. It is a normal part of life that should be embraced.

The False Teaching That Childbirth Is NOT Painful

Another lie to be wary of is that childbirth is not painful. I am here, as an older woman, who has birthed six children naturally, to tell you that birth is and will always be painful. It has been painful since creation.

God has predestined for us to have pain in childbirth. This is a hard word, isn't it? I know, I don't like it any more than you do; trust me. The truth about pain though, is that it always draws us to Him. He loves us so deeply that He wants us to hear His voice and know Him intimately.

It is not only extra-biblical, but also untrue to say that childbirth will not have some level of pain . . . in general. In Genesis 3, God spoke clearly to Adam and Eve as a Father in pain for His precious children who had sinned for the first time. Eve disobeyed God and broke His command to not eat from the Tree of the Knowledge of Good and Evil and then tempted Adam to do so. Adam sinned, eating of the fruit as well. The temptation and desire to be like God corrupted good judgment and over powered their discernment.

God punished Eve in Genesis 3:16. He said, "I will surely multiply your pain in childbearing; in pain you shall bring forth children." Not only was a woman's body created to give birth in pain, but after the fall, in "multiplied" pain. Childbirth is not easy, but He made us to be able to do it! And He promises to walk with us through it! Jesus Himself understands far greater pain and chose to undergo that for us so that we might live forever. We will discuss this topic of pain in childbirth much deeper in the chapters *Beautiful Pain, Understanding God's Design, 1 Timothy 2:15*, and *Fruitful Surrender*.

> "My son do not make light of the Lord's discipline, and do not lose heart when he rebukes you, because the Lord disciplines those He loves, and he punishes everyone he accepts as a son. Endure hardship as discipline; God is treating you as sons . . . God disciplines us for our good that we may share in his holiness. No discipline seems pleasant at the time, but painful. Later on however, it produces a harvest of righteousness and peace for those who have been trained by it." Hebrews 12:5-11, NIV

There are many books out there today that have helpful content, but some send the wrong message that if you are really spiritual you won't feel any pain in childbirth. If you feel pain, then you are doing it wrong, or you aren't reaching deep down enough into your spiritual self.

In Mark 13, Jesus is teaching His disciples about end times. He warns them (us), "Watch out that no one deceives you. Many will come in my name claiming, 'I am he,' and will deceive many. When you hear of wars and rumors of wars, do not be alarmed. Such things must happen, but the end is still to come. Nation will rise against nation, and kingdom against kingdom. There will be earthquakes in various places and famines. These are the beginning of birth pains. You must be on guard," (Mark 13:5-9, NIV).

> "Humble yourselves, therefore, under the mighty hand of God so that at the proper time he may exalt you, casting all your anxieties on him, because he cares for you. Be sober-minded; be watchful. Your adversary the devil prowls around like a roaring lion, seeking someone to devour. Resist him, firm in your faith, knowing that the same kinds of suffering are being experienced by your brotherhood [or sisterhood] throughout the world." 1 Peter 5:6-9

Ladies, God warns all believers to be on guard. We need to be careful that what we read on the topic of childbirth is not feeding us an extra-biblical or secular worldview. God created us, with all the necessary body gear to give birth. He created the birth process. What He created is good.

The Lord has likened birth pains and delivery to the process of the end of the world in this scripture. He says, "When you hear of wars and rumors of wars, do not be alarmed (nor should we dismay or 'be alarmed' in birth when we experience pain). Such things MUST happen, but the end (delivery/relief/salvation) is still to come." Why did the Lord liken end times to labor and childbirth? All throughout His-Story, women have given birth. In biblical days, before we had epidurals, all women had natural births. I am sure the cries of pain could be heard in the camps.

Men and women alike were aware of the pain, in one way or another. He knew people could relate to this analogy, this metaphor. Because birth was painful, but natural and necessary ... He was teaching that the process of getting to end times is also going to be painful, but necessary. He was teaching people to be aware of the trials, to be on guard and alert. In this same passage He warns his disciples they will be persecuted for their faith and brought before government officials. My fear is that in today's culture, where we have become desensitized to the sinfulness of this world, we have grown accustomed to excuses, and privileges. We are avoiding any painful consequences life might normally bring us because of our prosperity and blessings (in medicine, technology, and money) in this world. If we do not know the cost of pain in childbirth, what then is our lesson to heeding the Lord's warning?

What deceitful propaganda has crept into your belief system about childbirth?

To what degree would you say you have been influenced by this culture with regard to your beliefs, convictions, and dreams/visions of what you expect for your birth?

Lies and the Fears that Bind Us

When a woman finds out she is pregnant, a whole host of emotions, thoughts, and fears creep into her mind. While there is an initial response of excitement for most, usually following are fears of the unknown. Much of our culture portrays pregnancy and childbirth as ailments and burdens, rather than blessings. Because of the intimacy surrounding the topics of pregnancy, labor, and childbirth, many women do not grow up discussing this season in a woman's life from a confident or positive perspective.

Nevertheless, many young moms-to-be get their ideas of what to expect from the media, girlfriends, and unfortunately, most of what they hear does not promote having an intimate natural birth where they felt the Lord's presence. Thankfully, there are many helpful books available to expectant moms that help to ease some of the fears of pregnancy. To further exasperate our problems on the topic of pregnancy and birth, women today struggle with increasing physical challenges, such as more miscarriages, endometriosis, uterine and cervical cancer, and more infertility than any generation before us. ""About 10 % of women (6.1 million) in the United States ages 15–44 years have difficulty getting pregnant or staying pregnant."[7] The reality is today's women likely have friends or loved ones who have struggled with these health issues. Just getting pregnant and staying pregnant can be considered a challenge for many today.

As a pregnant woman, whether it is your first baby or your tenth, you will experience some form of fear at one time or another. Author Ina May

Gaskin writes, "The feelings of being overwhelmed, or feeling anxious, of not knowing what is best, of caring too much, of being inexperienced and inadequate are universal ones for all parents. In fact, the amount of anxiety that a new parent experiences may parallel just how much he or she cares about doing well by that baby."[8] Though these feelings, emotions, worries, and anxieties are universal, the truth that we as Christian women can cling to is that Jesus died for us to be free from these fears and worries when we trust in Him. Yes, it is natural and normal for us all to have times of worry and fear; we are human. But we as Christians have an advantage. We have the Lord, the Comforter, and our Creator, to whom we can go to with our fear and He will carry that burden. Dealing with our fears is part of the sanctifying process that comes with childbirth. If a woman can enter birth with no fear, her birth will go much faster. The truth is our fears hold us back physically and mentally in everything in life, including childbirth. Our fears, which are often created by lies we have come to believe or what we don't know, actually have the power to bind us. In childbirth, fear can actually slow down the progression of labor.

Why do I tell you this? Not to scare you more, but rather to bring to light the importance of dealing with fears. So that you can be motivated to clean out your mind of the lies and fears that prevent you from being and doing exactly what God intended for you. If you pursue truth with all your being—your heart, mind, soul, and strength—you will experience God more fully and experiencing Him in your birth, without burden or distraction of fear. God will reveal His truth to you and He will reveal His will for your birth.

I believe there is a misconception about fear among the church today, and this misconception greatly affects how we women deal with fear during childbirth. Many believe Jesus came in love so we would not fear God. They believe you cannot love God and fear Him at the same time. I have heard it stated that Jesus came to fill the gap that was created by fear. I believe it is critical that we address this, because as pregnant women in the body of Christ and as Titus 2 women who have had babies and are now mentoring younger women, the opportunity for addressing it is great. I believe Jesus came to bridge a gap in our union with God. We were separated from God because of our sinfulness and Jesus came to bridge the gap created by our sins by taking them away. Jesus came for us to have a relationship with Him. And in this relationship we may learn how to live more like Him, honoring the Father in how we live our lives, integrating our faith and relationship with Him into every area. Jesus came also to be our final sacrificial lamb. And as our final atonement, we can be free from the law of offering sacrifices. However, Jesus came to fulfill the law, not to expunge it. So It is important that we distinguish the differences between two biblical forms of fear—fear of God and fear of circumstances and people.

There are two kinds of fear, good fear that propels us toward obedience and blesses us with knowledge, wisdom and a closer relationship with God our Father, and fear that paralyzes us, consumes us, creates worry, and anxiety.

The Importance of Fearing of God

There are many more verses on the fear of the Lord. I would encourage you to do a word study on your own. (Deut. 6:13-16; Joshua 24:14-15; Psalm 2:11; Psalm 19:7-9; Prov. 1:7)

> *"The fear of the Lord is the beginning of wisdom; all those who practice it have a good understanding."*
> **Psalm 111:10**

When we as humble, finite humans have a correct theology and understanding of our mortality and abilities in comparison to God's infinite, immortal, omniscient, omnipotent headship, we can then have a fear of the Lord. Not a fear that separates us from knowing Him intimately, but a fear that puts Him on the pedestal He alone deserves, a pedestal no other human can attain. And

> *"Be not wise in your own eyes; fear the Lord and turn away from evil."*
> **Prov. 3:7**

it simultaneously humbles us to view ourselves in light of God's greatness. Simply put, understanding God helps us to hold Him in perspective to ourselves and builds unwavering love and respect for Him in our hearts.

Fearing God is the admittance of how powerful He is and the acknowledgement of how weak and unintelligent we are in comparison to Him. We need to have humble hearts toward our Creator and Father in heaven. It is when we have a healthy fear because we know what He is capable of doing and has done that we can respect Him for who He is. This knowledge brings us to His feet, on our knees, eager to learn from Him alone, eager to receive His Son, eager to trust Him to protect us. It humbles us to believe that, "I know nothing; God knows it all." And that belief makes us hungry for the Word of God, to glean His wisdom, His knowledge, His understanding, to follow His ways, and to keep His commandments. The more we are in the Word, the deeper our relationship with the Lord becomes and more our love for Him grows. Fearing God leads us to love and cherish Him more.

> "The fear of the Lord leads to life, and whoever has it rests satisfied; he will not be visited by harm." Prov. 19:23

> "And the Spirit of the Lord shall rest upon him, the Spirit of wisdom and understanding, the spirit of counsel and might, the Spirit of knowledge and the fear of the Lord. And his delight shall be in the fear of the Lord." Isaiah 11:2-3

A healthy fear of the Lord brings blessings, not curses. We as Christians today need to understand this fear is vital to our full relationship with God. Many cast out the teachings of the Old Testament, believing Jesus came to abolish the law, but He came to fulfill it. The Word of God stands true forever and endures forever.

The fear of the Lord brings us freedom not to fear the other fears our sin brings us and helps us to trust Him. "All you who fear the LORD, trust the LORD! He is your helper and your shield," (Psalm 115:11 NLT). When you fear the Lord, it is because you acknowledge His great power. His great power, once accepted, gives you a confidence not to fear all those other fears in life. You no longer fear circumstances, people, or death. You are set free from fear, when you put your trust in the One who is worthy of being feared.

> "Live as people who are free, not using your freedom as a cover-up for evil, but living as servants of God. Honor everyone. Love the brotherhood. Fear God. Honor the emperor." 1 Peter 2:16-17

Fear of Circumstances and People

The second type of fear is a fear that can consume, a fear that paralyzes and immobilizes us from the purposes for which we were created. These fears get to us when we don't have a healthy fear of the Lord, when we sin, or even just because we are human and we care too much about what man thinks. We sin when we start becoming self-consumed, thinking only of ourselves, thinking of our potential pain, it is even sin when we worry too much about our children

> *"But whoever listens to me will live in safety and be at ease, without fear of harm."*
> **Proverbs 1:33 (NIV)**

(creating anxiety). Ugly isn't it? Our fear reveals a lot about the condition of our hearts. I don't say this to condemn you, judge you, or make you feel inadequate. I struggle with giving fear the upper hand, allowing the enemy to use it to immobilize me at times. Like we discussed earlier, we all struggle with fear, which is why the Lord has addressed this issue so many times in the Bible. Fear is real. It happens to all of us. We fear people, judgment by others', failure, circumstances, pain and suffering, and we even fear the unknown.

For pregnant women, the temptation to fear is even more frequent as the D-day approaches. The anxiety that can accompany all the unknowns surrounding the labor and birth can be overwhelming, especially to a first-time mother. When a woman

> *"For I am the Lord, your God, who takes hold of your right hand and says to you, Do not fear; I will help you."*
> **Isaiah 41:13 (NIV)**

gets pregnant, often times the horror stories begin. Every woman who has given birth has a story to tell. Those who have experienced nightmare births have truly experienced a trauma in their lives. Talking about it with other women is one way they cope. When a woman shares her bad experience, often times it isn't intended to create fear in a new mother-to-be, rather it is to inform and warn her, but it is also her way of dealing with the trauma she went through. I believe most women do not intentionally want to scare other women or create more fears. Nonetheless, that is the outcome. The sad truth is many women do have bad birthing experiences.

I want to encourage you that God wants to redeem your childbirth. You can have an amazing experience.

The western culture's method of treating pregnancy and birth further exacerbates the potential fears. The message sent is that birth is an ailment or a disease, to be treated in the hospital, one with great pain and suffering, therefore, we should do our best to eliminate as much as pain as possible. Most of our culture believes the lie that women cannot birth babies safely unless they are in a hospital under the supervision of a medical professional. Decisions regarding the birth are then usually made based on these fears, information perceived through media, culture and friends, or education taught by professionals who hold to the belief that keeping medical control over the birth is better. Some even say to not have a baby in a hospital is irresponsible.

"Peace I leave with you; my peace I give to you. Not as the world gives do I give to you. Let not your hearts be troubled, neither let them be afraid" John 14:27

These convictions our culture teaches in the medical field stems from a deeper misguided belief that our bodies and our minds are not connected. In mainstream medicine, most doctors either treat mental illness (psychiatrists) or physical illness (physicians). The majority (not all) are not raised with a holistic viewpoint that all aspects of our bodies are connected.

"For God gave us a spirit not of fear, but of power and love and self-control." 2 Timothy 1:7

We as Christian women need to recognize we have been deceived; we have NOT been raised in a culture that views birth as a natural and normal life experience. Western medicine and media have dramatized birth to be perceived as a dangerous event that needs to be controlled. This leaves most women expecting not to have any choices other than to pick which hospital they want to have the baby at?

What we need is a complete overhaul of our mindset. We need to recognize our dilemma is not fearing the Lord, but rather avoiding the type of fear from those other things that He died to release us from. The fear of people (medical professionals or family members thinking we are crazy), what others may say, their opinions, fear of circumstances, and fears of the unknown. These fears are a reflection of something deeper within us. They are the inward emotion and anxiety that is triggered by an inaccurate view of birth and God's design of our bodies as women. Our fears are a reflection of a worldview that was taught to us our whole lives by our environment, our culture, and our experiences.

The beginning process for inviting God to redeem your birth begins as you allow Him to transform and renew your mind with regard to fear and your mindset of birth, by the washing of His word (see Romans 12). We need to recognize Jesus died for our fears, so we could live in freedom from fear.

After the fall, Adam and Eve hid from God. Why? Because they were afraid. Fear is something all people have dealt with, from the beginning, way back to the very first man and woman.

In Genesis 3:8-10, Adam and Eve "heard the sound of the Lord God walking in the garden in the cool of the day, and **the man and his wife hid themselves** from the presence of the Lord God among the trees of the garden. But the Lord God called to the man and said to him, 'Where are you?'

> *"I sought the Lord, and he answered me and delivered me from all my fears ... The angel of the Lord encamps around those who fear him and delivers them."*
> **Psalm 34:4,7**

And he said, 'I heard the sound of you in the garden, and **I was afraid** because I was naked, and **I hid** myself.'" (emphasis mine)

If you don't know the rest of the story I encourage you to go look it up. The reality of what happened is that Adam and Eve both sinned, they disobeyed God. It was because of their initial sin they became afraid. They had experienced an open and comfortable relationship with the Lord while being naked before they sinned. The key factor is their sin. So it is with us. In our sin, the sin of not acknowledging who God is and having a healthy fear of Him, we fail to trust Him to take care of us. In that sin, we fear death, and the trials of life's circumstances. In our sinful selfishness, we fear pain. We fear pain so much that we justify and rationalize why we don't deserve pain of any kind. Our culture, which thrives on self-indulgences, further justifies our selfish thinking. What we need is to realize our culture's worldview is not founded on the Word of

God nor belief in His design, His purposes, or following His will. And last of all, our culture is not about glorifying God—it is about glorifying self. We need to surrender our fears to Him. We need to live in the freedom of the cross. We need to turn from our sin, and run to our Father's arms. He is waiting to give us confidence, comfort, and healing.

Why is having a transformed mind with regard to fear so important in childbirth?

Our Fears Can Bind Us in Labor

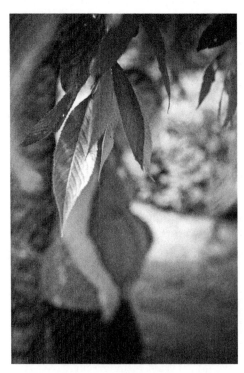

"For God has not given us a spirit of fear and timidity, but of power, love, and self-discipline." 2 Timothy 1:7, NLT

Our beliefs and fears can either slow down our labor, or help our labor progress at a more natural, uninhibited pace.

In Ina May's *Guide to Childbirth*, she gives examples of women who experience getting to a slower and stuck place in childbirth because of fears they had been dealing with or fears they had not dealt with. One such story is of a woman who was adopted and believed her biological mother had died while birthing her. Because of that belief, she feared she would die during childbirth as well and it caused her to experience some difficulties progressing while in labor. Gaskin writes,

"Once this profound fear was mentioned aloud, her cervix relaxed and displayed abilities it didn't possess earlier. It wasn't long before it was completely open. A healthy baby was born within two hours of the mention of the secret fear. I was quite impressed to know that an unspoken terrible thought could so powerfully alter a woman's body's ability to perform a normal physiological function. At the same time I was delighted to realize that a verbal solution to such a situation could remove any need for medication, mechanical intervention, or surgery."[9]

Another story explains a situation where, after many hours of unproductive labor, a birthing woman verbalized she feared her husband's lack of commitment to their relationship. Ina's husband then proceeded to have the couple repeat their marital vows. Within two hours of doing this, the baby was born.

"Every woman gets to a place during her [child] birth where she feels fearful, usually it happens just as the baby is about to come, during transition. Knowing this and anticipating this can give you power when you are in birth. You and your labor partner can prepare for this. When the time comes, speaking words of affirmation, reminding the birthing mother the baby is coming, is a powerful encouragement." Anonymous midwife

When my midwife shared this wisdom of observation with me, I took note to remember. Sure enough, as I was headed into transition, a fear started to creep into my mind that I couldn't do this (and this was my sixth baby). As I started to say, "I don't think . . . " I remembered what she told me and focused on the worship music playing in the background. I began to sing and believe the truth that God had designed my body to give birth. As I focused on the truth and not the lies and fears, I remember feeling the baby quickly moving down and my cervix opening. Within just a few minutes the baby was born.

There is a deep connection between our minds and our bodies.

In his book *Heaven*, Randy Alcorn states:

"As human beings, whom God made to be both physical and spiritual, we are not designed to live in a non-physical realm—indeed, we are incapable of even imagining such a place (or, rather, non-place). An incorporeal state is not only unfamiliar to our experience, but also incompatible with our God-given constitution. We are not, as Plato supposed, merely spiritual beings temporarily encased in bodies. Adam did not become a 'living being' – the Hebrew word *nephesh* – until he was both body and spirit (Genesis 2:7). We are physical beings as much as we are spiritual beings. That's why our bodily resurrection is essential to endow us with eternal righteous humanity, setting us free from sin, the Curse, and death."[10]

Our fears can affect our hearts, souls, our physical strength, and our minds with regard to obeying Him and doing what we were created to do. One function of the female's design is to carry and birth babies. When we fear what we were designed to do, sometimes that fear actually stops women from having children. A milder version is that when we fear what we were made to do, we try to take control over our circumstances. Ironically, taking control and not surrendering those fears is another example of what can bind a woman, preventing her from the physical ability to birth gently. The anxiety, the stress, and the fear can actually prevent labor from progressing, causing tension, because our thoughts (where our fears are created) directly impact our emotions (hormones) and our physical capacity to be open and relaxed. God designed our bodies so beautifully and intricately, able and ready to birth babies, but when we don't surrender and allow birth to happen naturally, it creates all kinds of stresses on our bodies, mentally, emotionally, physically, and spiritually. Many, not all, emergencies could be prevented if women would surrender their issues, their fears, their pasts, and their anxieties to God. Verbalizing these lies and fears can bring such relief, because we were not meant to carry our burdens alone. Verbalizing them can bring freedom from bondage. Once a woman is freed from her bondage and there is no more worry, she can focus on the task at hand, birthing her baby.

What are your fears? What lies have you believed that are preventing you from being able to fully embrace giving birth?

Another aspect of verbalizing fears and emotionally stressful issues that could have a massive impact on a woman's ability to focus on her birth would be pursuing reconciliation with friends or family members. During my sixth pregnancy, I was about ten days overdue and struggling with anxiety and fatigue from sleepless nights. There was tension between a family member and myself, and the stress was very overwhelming emotionally for me. As I was preparing spiritually and mentally for birth and seeking the Lord, I felt the Holy Spirit tugging at my soul to pursue truth and reconciliation in this relationship. Even though I knew this other person was not ready for reconciliation or hearing the truth, I pursued as directed by the Lord. Though it was extremely difficult and painful, and total reconciliation was not met during that meeting, I believe the freedom that came from simply pursuing reconciliation, simply getting feelings off my chest, and staying true to myself before God, speaking truth in love, is what allowed me peace in my soul. Ultimately that peace that comes from releasing a burden helped me focus on the Lord and get ready to give birth. I had no sorrow in the back of my mind, no distraction from this restless turmoil within a dear relationship of mine.

Coincidentally, I went into labor the very next morning and experienced a speedy, yet perfectly engaged birth. I had no thoughts holding me back from what I was called to focus on. I am so thankful to God for speaking to me and giving me the confidence to step out in faith and pursue healing in this way.

God began a process of redeeming a relationship in my life and one of blessings that came from dealing with those emotions before birth was a focused and peaceful birth, devoid of tension, and with reduced pain. I was able to focus on Jesus, to seek Him with no distractions. I was able to surrender fully to the Lord and what He created my body to do. I focused my mind on Jesus and told myself to surrender as I sang "I Surrender All" in labor.

When you focus on the Lord and not the things of this earth, nor the angst of the moment, you transcend above the pain. In just a moment of losing focus on Jesus, you begin to start thinking of yourself and your pain, and the pain gets more intense. As you think about the pain of each contraction, you begin to digress in your belief that you can actually do it. The further your focus away from the Father, the less confident you'll feel and the more you will focus on the pain. You cannot focus on the things of this earth at the same time as focusing on the things above. In Colossians, God gives us a command to focus on Him, on things above (heaven) and not on the things of this earth. This is key to experiencing the presence of the Lord in birth. The more you obey this command the less you are in pain. You simply cannot focus on your pain, while focusing on God.

"Since, then, you have been raised with Christ, set your hearts on things above, where Christ is, seated at the right hand of God."

Colossians 3:1 (NIV)

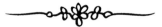

"No temptation has overtaken you that is not common to man. [The temptation to fear the what ifs in regard to childbirth is common to women] God is faithful, and he will not let you be tempted beyond your ability, but with the temptation he will also provide the way of escape, that you may be able to endure it [Focusing on Him is our escape, it is how we can endure]." 1 Corinthians 10:13

In His book, *Heaven,* Randy Alcorn also states:

> "The command to think about heaven is under attack in a hundred different ways every day. Everything militates against it. Our minds are so much set on Earth that we are unaccustomed to heavenly thinking. So we must work at it . . . . C.S. Lewis

observed, 'If you read history, you will find that the Christians who did most for the present world were just those thought most of the next . . .' We need a generation of heavenly minded people who see human beings and earth itself not simply as they are, but as God intends them to be."[11]

We as women can expect and anticipate there will be times of fear, worry, and doubt coming our way when we become pregnant with a child. In those times, we can choose to surrender those fears to Jesus and allow Him to redeem them, rather than letting them consume us and affect how we make decisions in childbirth.

Live victoriously. Jesus died once and for all so we wouldn't have to carry those burdens. We may have moments of physical weakness, when we are tempted to rely on our own strength and fail. We may have moments when we struggle to hold it together emotionally because we lack self-control (a fruit of the Spirit) and then we fall to sin. We may have those moments when we fear and get overwhelmed with anxiety because we are not trusting in the Lord enough. We need to anticipate these fears will be our spiritual challenges as we run the race as Christians. Does that mean we just allow them to dictate our growth and what we do in life?

The fears you and I face with regard to pregnancy and birth are common to all women. We need to anticipate the challenges before they come, and prepare for whatever the Lord has for us. Knowing we can expect these emotions and fears when pregnant gives us the edge. Allow Jesus to complete a work in you that He started and finished when He died on the cross for your sins. Just as He stood up to the enemy when Satan tempted Him in the desert after He was baptized, we need to stand up to Satan. These fears, feelings of inadequacy, are universal, but Jesus died for these. He makes us whole.

The victory is ours as Christians. When we call out our fears and take them to the Lord in order to have victory over them, we are winning a battle against Satan and the power he is battling to have over us. He does not want us to live in the freedom Christ died for. He wants us to be oppressed. He doesn't want us to live joyful, productive lives that glorify our Father in heaven. He wants us to be consumed with fear and be handicapped, or worse, paralyzed, so we are immobilized warriors. This fear of circumstances, of the unknown, is natural; it is our human nature. Knowing that all humans struggle with that same challenge should empower you to move toward seeking freedom from the bondage of fear. God does not want us to fear circumstances, mankind, or the what ifs.

Learning how to battle this fear in preparing for childbirth and while in birth is the perfect boot camp for motherhood as well. When you win the battle, with the Lord's help, and you cry out victory with a healthy beautiful baby in your arms, there is nothing more powerful in the world. The confidence you have in Christ is set in stone, your journey of faith is so much stronger, and you are more equipped for all the hard decisions and the laboring in love you will continue to do the rest of your life. Embrace it!

Fears Experienced in Pregnancy & Childbirth

First Trimester Fears
About the baby

Am I going to be a good parent? Will I fail my baby? Will I miscarry the baby? Will the baby be healthy?

As far as being a good parent goes, God chose you to be your baby's mother. He handpicked you. If you allow God to mold you, to refine you through the journey of parenting, then no one on earth is more equipped than you to raise your child. We cannot do well at anything on our own. We need Jesus to forgive us and sanctify us, and we need the Holy Spirit to guide us. Without His influence in our lives, we cannot be good parents on our own. None of us can. I have failed mine many times. It is a good thing we don't have to be perfect. We are to strive to be imitators of Christ. He knows we cannot be Him. But with God, you will be the perfect parent for your child; that is why God chose you.

Having a miscarriage is a normal and common fear for many women, especially with the rate of miscarriages today. All you can do is take care of yourself, get plenty of rest, have faith in Him, and pray. Leave it up to the Lord. These things are beyond our control.

Babies are made by God and are unique just the way God intended them to be. Our inability to look at ourselves the way God does can make us more fearful about whether our babies fall within normal standards. But God doesn't view disabilities or differences like we do. Don't fret about specific health issues in general, because it creates a massive stress on you and your baby. Know that He creates every person different from others and just right in His sight.

Focus on trusting God. Study more about dealing with fear in Scripture. Pray with your husband, a mentor, or your mother. Find someone you can sit and talk with in prayer about your fears. Verbalize and give them to God, trusting in Him.

Marital Fears

Are we ready to have a baby? A baby is a big responsibility. Can we afford it or will it put stress on us? Will my husband still want to have sex with me while I am pregnant, and if he doesn't, is he going to leave me?

These fears can consume couples throughout pregnancy. While you are thinking a baby is a big responsibility, your husband is probably thinking about how much money a baby will cost. While you are upset about sexual intimacy, I guarantee he is upset about it as well. This is a time when you both need to talk and keep open communication, especially about fears. When it comes to sex, you or your husband may have fears about hurting the baby. Feeling timid about those topics might prevent them from being communicated. Go the distance and try to be transparent. It will only strengthen your marriage. If you have fears your husband is going to leave you, then you really need to go on a date with him and have a serious talk, sharing your fears. If you have legitimate fears I would suggest finding a Christian counselor in your church.

Health Related Concerns

In the first trimester, women can have a host of different pregnancy symptoms, from intense morning sickness, to chronic fatigue, to hormonal imbalances leading to depression. All of these symptoms and more add to the emotional and hormonal changes pregnant women experience, often furthering fears. If not dealt with, these symptoms can create more issues that can lead to deeper fears when the day of delivery approaches.

On the other hand, there are many women who have blessed pregnancies. Physically they feel great. They have no problem keeping up their normal pace. Some work all the way through their pregnancies, up until the day before. They seem to have a glow and energy about them. The unfortunate thing for some, but not all, of these women can come if they have unresolved fears and issues that don't come out in the first trimester, but later, during the birth process, causing the slow, prolonged labor that comes from stress, worry, and fear. If they have not dealt with physical stress, fatigue, pain, or suffering until the last stage of labor it can be hard for these women because they have missed out on the "boot camp" stage of morning sickness and chronic fatigue that ease you into what may come later. (This isn't true of all; it is a POTENTIAL issue for some.)

Second Trimester Fears & Issues

As pregnancy progresses and women's bellies start showing, what should be excitement instead brings on a whole host of body image issues for women that, for some, they haven't ever dealt with before. When it comes time to buy maternity clothes, this can oftentimes be the first financial stress on couples. While the woman desires to feel beautiful for her husband, sometimes the finances just aren't available and need to be saved for when the baby arrives. The phrase "mama always comes last," begins to become a reality, as there are so many expenses with a new baby on the way. Most often Mommy does not have much of a budget for clothing for herself. Self-esteem can be greatly affected during pregnancy, especially for women who didn't have a secure sense of body image before they were pregnant.

In this trimester, as the woman begins to show more, physical intimacy between husband and wife can change greatly due to fears of hurting the baby, which are perfectly normal for both husband or wife to have. This insecurity can further exacerbate the body image issue for them.

Third Trimester Fears

By the third trimester, sleepless nights begin, and so does the tendency to be more emotional and cranky. This can add extra stress on the marriage relationship. Every woman's body is different. Some women experience a heightened desire for intimacy, while others can experience pain during intercourse. All these factors play into the heart and emotions of a woman as the day of delivery draws near.

Fears about Pain

As the day approaches, doubts about handling the pain of childbirth begin to sneak into expectant mothers' minds. They wonder if they will be fully ready and able to deliver the child naturally and they worry about the severity of the pain.

In Isaiah 14:3 it says, "On the day the Lord gives you relief from suffering and turmoil and cruel bondage." (NIV) It is true that birth is painful, but in that pain God can show Himself merciful; He can show you relief through His supernatural power and strength.

Fear about circumstances and people

Some women worry about whether they chose the right birth/labor partners were the right choice? (Should they have asked them?) Others are taunted by all the things that could go wrong at the birth (all the what ifs).

What if I have to have a caesarean? What will people think of me? Well, if you experience an emergency that endangers your life or the baby's, then you may have to have a caesarean. Will you love your baby any less? Of course not. Let's choose NOT to fear things, but instead get educated, and then trust in the Lord. If you focus on trusting Him and you have a caesarean, you will get through it. God will give you all you need to get through what you experience. In the meantime, focus on the truth that God designed your body to do this. Anticipate the good; don't focus on the fears. You could potentially create your worst nightmare simply by stressing yourself out so much that your physiological responses may be dictated by your fear. So focus on the Lord.

Fears about Death

What if I die? What if my baby dies?

Many women fear death in birth. Why? Because a woman who is pregnant is faced, sometimes for the first time, with her mortality. As humans we need to be humble in acknowledging we are not immortal, and the experience of giving birth naturally can be one of those instances in life that bring you closer to that reality. It can forever imprint in your mind the reality of our humanity and the need for a Savior.

We need to have a healthy realization of our mortality, but we must also have a growing trust in the Lord and His will for our lives.

Do you fear dying?

David feared dying. In Psalm 55:4-5, "My heart is in anguish within me; the terrors of death have fallen upon me. Fear and trembling come upon me, and horror overwhelms me."

Come to the Lord. Ask Him. Wait on Him. Let Him show you His mercy. Don't hide from your fear. Verbalize it as David did when he cried out to God. Cry out to God. He wants you to cry out to Him and to embrace you and show you how merciful He is. "Be merciful to me, O God, be merciful to me, for in you my soul takes refuge; in the shadow of your wings I will take refuge, till the storms of destruction pass by. I cry out to God Most High, to God who fulfills his purposes for me," (Psalm 57:1-2).

A friend of mine, Amber, shared some beautifully God honoring insights as she prepared her heart to receive another blessing from the Lord. We can all relate and learn from what the Lord has been teaching her through her childbearing years:

"The daunting concept of giving birth, especially giving birth naturally, can be a frightening thing to ponder. Even on the verge of having my fifth baby, I'm still afraid when I think of it; "Yikes, I have to do it again?" There's just no way around it! Thankfully, God in His mercy decided to bless us with another child. I don't want another c-section, and I'd prefer to not have any interventions that might lead to one, so I just have to go through it. It's like walking through a door of fear, and even though I know there's the joy of having my baby on the other side, nothing in me wants to do it. Just prior to my fourth birth, I was talking to my husband about this fear, and he graciously reminded me that, though I'm afraid to walk through that door, I do not walk through it alone. Jesus Christ is walking through it with me. And it is HE who will deliver this child. No one else but Jesus is more capable to empathize with my fearful expectation of the pain in front of me, with my suffering, and with the indescribable joy of birthing new life on the other side (see John 16:21, Isaiah 53:10-11, Hebrews 12:2, Hebrews 2:10-18). And since all fear is ultimately rooted in the fear of death and Jesus OVERCAME death for me, I have nothing to fear when He is present with me."

The anxiety and fear we experience during pregnancy can emotionally, physically, and spiritually impact our perspectives and expectations for our birth experiences. Amber learned that "Jesus would walk closely with her through the anxieties and pain of labor, and that He understood intimately what she was feeling. He would strengthen her to face her fears and overcome them in His name." This truth, which she so eloquently shares is for all who will call upon the name of Jesus Christ, "casting all your anxieties on him, because he cares for you." (1 Peter 5:7, ESV)

Our Fears Are a Temptation

The temptation is to carry our own burdens and to withhold from God, others, and ourselves. The reality is when we do not face our fears and choose to give them to God, we are choosing to live in bondage. We are choosing not to receive the mercy Jesus already died to give us. That mercy comes in the form of freedom. You can experience freedom when you are not oppressed by fear. Satan tempted Jesus to betray God after fasting in the desert for forty days. I think he knew that because Jesus was human He would be physically weak. It was the perfect time to tempt Him in the enemy's eyes. When you are in bondage and living in fear, you are weak. In your weakness, you are more likely to fall to temptation.

"Cast your cares on the LORD and he will sustain you; he will never let the righteous fall."
Psalm 55:22 (NIV)

If you are planning to pursue a natural birth, and your heart's desire is to serve God, be a light that shines for Jesus by worshipping Him and praising Him while in labor. If you are planning to invite the presence of the Lord into your birth, I guarantee you will be tempted. The enemy will tell you lies. Lies such as, "you can't do this" and "you are too weak". Do you know why Satan wants you to believe his lies and alter your birth decisions? He doesn't want you to grow in the Lord. He doesn't want you to be blessed by your birth experience. He doesn't want you to tell other people about the miracles of God and how real He is. He doesn't want you to experience God in this intimate way. He doesn't want your marriage to grow. He doesn't want your family to be strengthened. He doesn't want you to tell other people about this blessing in birth. He doesn't want God glorified in the hospitals. He doesn't want God glorified in front of midwives. This is a spiritual battle. So be on guard of the enemy. He will send his message many ways. Sometimes even through those close to you or doubters who have believed his lies and fallen to this temptation of fear. Stay focused and alert. Be in the Word of God so you can discern the devil's schemes.

"Delight yourselves in the Lord, and he will give you the desires of your heart."
Psalm 37:4

> "He himself likewise partook of the same things . . . and delivered all those who through fear of death were subject to lifelong slavery . . . For because he himself has suffered when tempted, he is able to help those who are being tempted." Hebrews 2:14-15, 18
>
> ———⌇———
>
> "For we do not have a high priest who is unable to sympathize with our weaknesses, but one who in every respect has been tempted as we are, yet without sin. Let us then with confidence, draw near to the throne of grace, that we may receive mercy and find grace to help in time of need."
> Hebrews 4:15-16

Jesus knows our struggles; He partook of the same things and has given us victory over those fears. He has delivered us. Isn't there a beautiful imagery in being delivered from our fears and our sins, and the gift we have to be able to experience delivering our children in the flesh? God is so good to us that He has given us this privilege to know Him more intimately through this act of deliverance.

Deliverance from Fears

Jesus models a path to deliverance from these fears for us

We are in a battle to live in the freedom that Jesus Christ died for. Freedom from fears that disable us from living the life we were meant to live. We need to not only recognize this battle, but also take up the armor in the Word of God in Ephesians 6 and choose to walk in the faith that comes from understanding the word of God. We have an enemy that has deceived us and used fear as a main tool to distract us, discourage us, and disable us from experiencing the fullness of Christ and His spiritual blessings in many areas of our lives.

Satan does not want strong Christian couples having babies and raising them for the glory of God. The reality is that he will try his best to discourage you and make your experience one that you are not willing to experience again in order to bring forth life.

If we acknowledge this challenge and we proclaim the Holy Scriptures as we fight the good fight to live in faith and not fear we can overcome his attacks on the family and on marriage today. We can choose to allow God to redeem our hard situations for His good.

1) Verbalize your fears to close friends or family who love you and will pray with you.

When Jesus Himself was "greatly distressed" (Mark 14:33) and "very sorrowful, even to death" (Matthew 26:38), His closest disciples were chosen to accompany Him. They failed and fell asleep on the job. Then He came back and said, "Are you asleep? Watch and pray that you may not enter into temptation. The spirit indeed is willing, but the flesh is weak" (Matthew 26:38-41). Jesus knew His disciples were going to become fearful of being called followers of Jesus. He warned Peter he would deny Him three times before the rooster crowed. He knew the temptation was great because the disciples would fear for their own lives once they saw Him arrested, condemned, and tortured. He knew that temptation full well, because He himself was distressed, troubled, and sorrowful, even to death. However, He still asked them to go with Him, to "keep watch with him." He didn't want to be alone.

In your fear, seek out other strong Christian women and talk to your husband. Tell them your fears. Let them pray for you. Let them "keep watch with you." Those people will be assets in your labor in holding you accountable to NOT fear but to let God carry it. They can encourage you with words, Scriptures, and prayer while you labor. They will say what you need to hear to let this fear go, but you need to be vulnerable and real with them.

2) Go to God in prayer; submit your will to Him as Jesus did unto the Father.

"And he withdrew from them about a stone's throw, and knelt down and prayed, saying 'Father, if you are willing, remove this cup from me. Nevertheless, not my will, but yours be done.' And there appeared to him an angel from heaven, strengthening him. And being in agony he prayed more earnestly; and his sweat became like great drops of blood falling to the ground," (Luke 22:41-44). Jesus gave His life completely to His Father in heaven. God answered His prayer by sending an angel to strengthen Him. While Jesus was in agony, He prayed more and He had physical expressions of severe pain—He sweat drops of blood. Our human bodies are not meant to handle the intense stress of fearing death. Now Jesus knew the upcoming torture was going to kill Him. He knew His closest disciples would fall to sin and hide. He had much more pain and fear than you or I could ever possibly imagine, but He gave us a model to follow—to ask others to carry our burden with us, to pray for us, and then to cry out to God in prayer.

What Is Fear of Death Really?

Fearing death really shows a love for our own lives! Yucky isn't it? Our selfishness is blatantly clear. "Whoever loves his life loses it, and whoever hates his life in this world will keep it for eternal life," (John 12:25). We

> *"Because he loves me, says the Lord, I will rescue him; I will protect him, for he acknowledges my name."*
> Psalm 91:14, NIV

need to be completely surrendered to God, trusting that He knows what is best for us and He will provide it. When we worry and fear for our lives, we selfishly love our lives more than we trust that God is really in control and that His power and will is sufficient. As mothers there is another reality as to why we fear dying, isn't there? It may not be at all that we personally fear death, but that we understand the immense responsibility we have to raise our children. Even though that is a sign of our love for our children, it is also a reflection of how much we trust God to take care of them even better than we ever could.

This is a universal truth for all humankind. We all struggle with loving our own lives and not fully trusting God's will for our lives. Maybe not all in the same circumstances, but we do.

Learning to trust isn't ever easy, but trusting in the Lord is what gives you courage not to fear!

When I was pregnant with my sixth child, I had terrible morning sickness and other health and back related issues. At eleven weeks gestation I was hospitalized for a week and then on bed rest for two months. While in the hospital, we were advised by doctors to consider terminating our pregnancy. Of course aborting was never an option in our minds. Sadly though, it was amazing how many people around us questioned our decisions. You see, I had a very hard pregnancy with my fifth baby as well and was on semi-bed rest for six weeks. Because of what I had gone through, many people questioned why we would ever have more children. My thought process was not on myself. My husband and I had taken it to the Lord as we did every time, and asked Him to lead us in our decision either way. We felt strongly the Lord had blessed us with this child for a reason. I knew in my heart there must be a large calling on his life if Satan already wanted him dead. You see we are in a battle, many battles today. As Christians, we need to fight the good fight and in doing so be willing to get some skinned knees and hurt feelings.

I had to deal with the reality that I might not ever walk again and that scared me. I had to wrestle with the Lord again, like I did when I found a benign tumor on the side of my face. I yelled and cried. I got angry and wrestled with Him (in a hospital bed, of course). But that was when God provided the strength and words of affirmation to me through the people who were seeking Him and hearing Him. He used older women who had gone before me to encourage me. The Body of Christ was His hands, His feet, His mouth, His shoulders, and His heart. They spoke His truth to me when I was frustrated, confused, and hurting. Why do I share this with you? Because God taught me something in all of these hard trials that happen in life. He taught me His faithfulness. He taught me about His mercy. He taught me more about grace. And even though I still have a lot to learn, I wouldn't trade any of the experiences I had—even the darkest moments, because they have made me who I am today and have molded my faith to be what it is. Those experiences put me on the path of learning from God how to live for Him more, and my life is bright because of Him.

During this pregnancy I had endured severe morning sickness, a herniated bulging disc in my back and other spinal issues, hospitalization, bed rest, and all the emotional and relational ups and downs that come with such an intense situation as I found myself in. Throughout my pregnancy, I dealt with depression, feeling like I was a failure and listening to the lies this world indoctrinates into people's minds. I was doing my best, but constantly dealt with people questioning why we were having more children. Everyone had an opinion as to what God's will for our family was, but I was trying desperately not to listen to them and to hear the voice of the one true God.

During the time I was on bed rest, I began getting feeling back in my legs and my morning sickness got more bearable. As I went to my prenatal appointments with my midwives at the local water birth center, they suggested I also meet with a midwife at the local hospital in case my condition or the baby's took a turn for the worse as was predicted by the neurologist and osteopath. Their belief was that I needed to schedule a cesarean in order to avoid potential spinal surgery. Trusting their medical advice, I pursued both avenues for the remainder of my last two trimesters, but began feeling stronger and stronger as the final months neared. I kept doing my water therapy, which included exercises to strengthen my back, and found I felt the strongest while I was in the water. In my final months of appointments with the specialists, they all agreed that a miracle had occurred in my back, but out of precaution felt strongly that I should still schedule a cesarean.

I was at a crossroads. On one hand, I had dreamt and planned my birth and knew what my heart longed for with my husband there by my side, my girls there as well worshiping with me as we welcomed another little Tolpin into the world. On the other hand, I didn't want to be foolish or prideful just because I had had five other great births. I knew we (Isaac and I) had to make the decision, but what I really wanted was for God to be clear with me about what His will was for me and my family. As I sought Him in prayer, through meditation of the Word, and a whole lot of worship, I felt the Lord telling me not to make a decision in fear. I was leaning toward the hospital birth because I was scared, even after all He had done for me so far. He had taken my broken, hurting body and allowed me to heal and my baby to grow stronger inside my womb, protected and safe, despite the medications I had taken to stop the vomiting. Why wouldn't I trust Him? As the days came nearer and nearer, I grew stronger in my conviction of having the baby as planned at the birth center, I had a peace about it. I had no fear.

I knew in my heart I needed to simply listen to what the Lord's will was for my baby and me. In any other circumstance I believe I would have chosen the hospital, but I felt the Lord asking me to trust Him. I felt God was testing my faith and I wanted so badly to please and trust Him. My husband and I prayed about this decision a lot over the course of my pregnancy. In prayer we felt confident to have the baby at the water birth center. I am not advocating that this is the course of action everyone should take. I am simply sharing a story of God's faithfulness in my life and how He had mercy on me after all I had endured. I believe strongly that every woman/couple should make a decision as to where they should birth their baby based on their own personal convictions and what they feel the Lord is impressing on their hearts for their families, in their particular situations.

God's Mercy in Ethan's Birth

After weeks of feeling like a ticking time bomb the day finally arrived. As the Sunday morning bustle commenced, I focused inward, trying to read my body. Was this the big day? Kids showering, getting all cleaned up for church, packing bags, and all the usual details of the morning, but with added pleasure of grandma's company. As Grandma Sarah (my mother-in-law) and my husband Isaac held down the fort, I went for a little walk out in the vineyard and around the property. It was a beautiful day and I seemed to notice more of God's beauty than usual. Even the weeds looked extra healthy, and I didn't mind; instead I marveled. As I walked, I would stop every few minutes to focus. I still wasn't positive if I was going into labor. After all, I had been dilated for weeks, and for the first time in all my pregnancies, I was overdue. I was certain the baby was going to be huge. My last two were in the high nine pounds and they were early and on time. A natural fear entered my mind for an instant, what if this baby is eleven pounds and posterior again? Then as I kept walking, a song entered my heart, "Deliverer" by Vicky Beeching. The fear subsided and I felt strong. I had a confidence the Lord would be my strength, even if I had none. I had been down this road and had known God to be faithful and strong, but I still had a hint of fear: *what if?*

I called my midwife, Adele, and talked to her as Isaac was loading the kids to go to church. At that point I wasn't having regular contractions, but I was feeling pressure and it was coming and going in waves like contractions. Adele was on her way to church so she told me to text her with updates. Just ten minutes later I was texting her, "This is the real deal, meet you at birth center." As the kids were riding bikes outside and enjoying time with grandma before she was going to head back home, I felt an urgency to get to the birth center. Things began to progress quickly within the next fifteen minutes. Isaac, Kelsey, and I headed for the water birth center while Sarah waited for Keziah (our awesome friend and helper) to stay with Luke and Drew. Then once Keziah arrived to take care of the little ones at home, Gramma Sarah brought Austin and Megan to meet us.

Once we got to the birth center things started to speed up fast. We had enough time to settle in and get my birth music playing.

I reminisced as I thought through my last births for a moment, drawing strength from those victories in the Lord. Each of my births was an amazing experience, each one unique. This birth, though, was different in that I really met the Lord of mercy. The Almighty was gracious to me and had mercy on me. He heard my cries during my pregnancy and He blessed me. He knew the desire of my heart was to glorify Him in all things. He chose me to mother and raise this child, for that I am eternally grateful. The Lord knew my heart to glorify and magnify Him in labor and delivery that I might pass on a strong legacy to my daughters and my son who were there.

Kelsey and Megan were both in the room with us and got to participate in the labor and delivery. Austin was there for most of the time. He went out when I first got in the tub and then waited in the family area with grandma and one of our other friends, Kirsten. They all came in right after the baby was born and Austin met his new baby brother. I can't tell you how special it was to have my daughters there with me. Megan (five years) had her hand on my shoulder, and Kelsey (ten) still timing and offering homeopathy loved being a part of the process. To have them singing and worshipping with me and witnessing the birth of Ethan was an experience I look back on with so much delight.

Isaac was a gentle but strong man during this birth. He was my main coach. Together we birthed this baby as he gently swayed me in his strong arms as I lay on him. He came in the tub and held me up so I could float and stretch. I am certain this added in relieving pain in my back, as well as speeding up the process of birth. When contractions got more intense, he changed the intensity, rocking me harder, back and forth. Without communicating, he simply just followed his instincts and heart to serve me and follow what my body was doing. We raised hands in worship to the Lord through each contraction. As I reached the self-denial stage (in transition), I faced it head on for what it was. Knowing all women go through it, I remembered what my midwives told me, "That is when the baby is about to come." I focused on the promise to come in my son. Anticipating his arrival, helped me to focus, and soon thereafter he was born. I remember thinking later that my husband just rocked that baby right out of me. Ethan descended so quickly that I can truthfully say it was one of the easiest births even though he was 9 lbs. 1 oz. Isaac delivered Ethan . . . the first one he personally delivered and he did a great job. We enjoyed hanging out in the tub for about forty minutes, just praying and embracing the moment.

Ethan was born in one hour and forty-five minutes from the time we got to the water birth center. His birth was the second fastest of all my births, but it was exhilarating. After his birth the first thing I cried out was "The Lord had mercy on your mother!" I meant it. I was amazed; my back didn't hurt during the delivery at all. That was a new experience for me. In my mind it was my perfect birth. I praise God almighty for his strength, nurturing, and mercy.

I would like to share the lyrics to the song that Ethan was born to. My children all have birth songs. It is so special for me to remember their births when I hear these songs . . . it brings back the beautiful memories of these most spiritual times in my life. In my mind, the birth experience is the only experience in a woman's life that can challenge her so deeply, physically, mentally, spiritually, and emotionally. It affects the mind, body and soul in a way like no other. My heart has always been to purposefully dedicate this event in my life to Jesus and invite Him to be present and in charge.

Ethan's Birth Song

Here are some of the lyrics to the song that was playing when I delivered Ethan and the few minutes afterward.

Depth of Mercy
By Selah

"Depth of mercy can there be
Mercy still reserved for me?...

Heaven find me on my knees
Hear my soul's impassioned plea

There were moments I remember singing this song in labor and being deeply moved, and then moments when I was so focused I don't remember the words but I was at peace.

Then, as Ethan was born, I was so moved by how the Lord spared me pain in my back, which is truly a miracle and testimony to His power, empathy to pain, and mercy.

My prayer is that as Ethan grows—like the lyrics in this song profess—Ethan would be "inclined to repent" and "weep, believe, and sin no more." That Ethan would have the kind of communion with the Lord I have been so grateful to experience. That the Lord would hear his "soul's impassioned plea."

Mercy was reserved for me and is for you as well!

God was so gracious to me in letting me enjoy my last few months and delivering me from most of my pain. Every day, I had little reminders of my immortality as I dealt with pains in my back, but overall God had been so merciful. I think I subconsciously thought I had used up whatever mercy He had for me during my pregnancy. Why do I say this? Because as I prepared my mind for a longer birth, God blessed me again and granted me an easier labor and delivery. Just because He can. He is that good. I knew without a doubt I did not deliver my baby. The Lord delivered him.

Our God is a great God and has the power to bless His children with unlimited healing, unlimited mercy, and boundless protection and safety! God used this experience in my life to teach me about Himself, His mercy and His faithfulness.

So as you prepare for your birth, examine your heart, check your thoughts and beliefs. Be real with your husband and labor partners. Don't let fear tempt you to sin in your relationship with the Lord by not trusting Him. Don't withhold from Him. Don't let fear ruin your birth. "Pray and watch that you not be tempted." Let us draw near to Him who understands, offers counsel, confidence, and deliverance.

Let God's will be done in your life by submitting your plans to Him. We are not to fear circumstances, but in all things focus on Him who is our hope, in Him whom we can trust because He will never let us go and He will never fail us.

> *"Who shall separate us from the love of Christ? Shall trouble or hardship or persecution or famine or nakedness or danger or sword? As it is written: 'For your sake we face death all day long; we are considered as sheep to be slaughtered.' No, in all these things we are more than conquerors through him who loved us. For I am convinced that neither death, nor life, neither angels nor demons, neither the present nor the future, nor any powers, neither height nor depth nor anything else in all creation, will be able to separate us from the love of God that is in Christ Jesus our Lord." Romans 8:35-39 (NIV)*

> *"I consider that our present sufferings are not worth comparing with the glory that will be revealed in us."*
> *Romans 8:18 (NIV)*

Pray with me

Lord, deliver us from the fear of circumstances, the unknown, and the fear of people. Please help us surrender our fears to You. Give us courage to obey You and take action in facing our fears and dealing with them, whatever they may be. Help us to love and yearn for holiness and for living in freedom from the bondage that fear can cripple us with.

If someone who is reading this is in need of reconciling past hurts in a relationship so she can be freed from the bondage that conflict creates and to live without anxiety and stress, please give her courage and perseverance to see it through.

Savior, we are all guilty of loving our own lives too much at one point or another. We ask You to forgive us for our selfishness in loving ourselves too much. Please help us to love You and Your ways more than ourselves. Help us to surrender all to You and live what we believe, which is that we were created not to fulfill our own desires, but for much greater things that glorify you. May we pursue living lives worthy of the cross and with sincerity of heart pursue living in relationships with our brothers and sisters in Christ with transparency and humility, thinking not too highly of ourselves, but in compassion putting one another's needs above our own.

Help us to focus on you and not on earthly things. Protect our minds and hearts from being deceived by any of this world's message that is not in alignment with Yours. Give us discernment and wisdom. Equip us with the strength of mind and passion of heart to do Your will and oppose beliefs that are not of You. Let us live our lives pursuing You and peace in all we do. Grant us peace of heart, mind, and soul so we can be focused on You in childbirth, not distracted by any lies or fears. Help us to make our decisions based on truth, not fears. Thank You, Jesus, for dying so we can live in freedom from the bondage of sin. Help us not to sin against You in making idols or allowing anything to consume our thoughts and hearts that are not of You.

We love You, Lord, for what You have done, what You are doing, and what You are going to do. We love You for who You are. May we know You more intimately as we seek to surrender all to You and experience Your presence in our lives, in our joys and blessings and in our sufferings and trials. To You be the glory for the great things You have done.

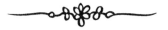

Part III

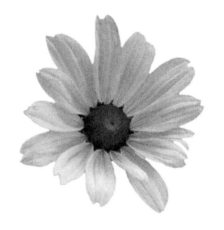

Embracing His Miracle

The statement, "embracing God's miracle" encompasses many things, including:

- Accepting the reality and blessing of parenthood
- Marveling in the miraculous creation of your sweet baby and having confidence in God's design of your body to nurture and bring forth life
- Understanding that this is His miracle and submitting your will under His authority
- Attesting to the purpose behind the pain
- Experiencing life's blessings, trials, and sufferings in total surrender, with a teachable heart
- Appreciating your husband and those laboring with you, leaning on them and growing in your relationships because you are sharing this experience
- Holding your precious sweet baby for the first time in your arms, delighting in his/her presence

When someone embraces another spiritually, there is acceptance and sincerity of heart, mind, and soul. Anyone can hug another physically, but to *embrace* another requires a depth of intention and acceptance. The intimate experience of childbirth is one where there is an opportunity for a sincere embrace to impact many lives. When a mother and daughter literally embrace one another, laboring together, there is a newer and stronger bond formed. The marriage relationship also can be strengthened in ways like no other because wife and husband are engaged together, as a team, embracing one another and working together to bring forth their new child. In labor and delivery, embracing this experience as God's miracle can empower the woman to be strong. It can be what she needs when her strength is gone to move beyond any lies or fears. An embrace of a like-minded labor partner who can remind the laboring mother-to-be whose power she can rely on is revolutionary.

To surrender one's birth to the Lord, allowing Him to redeem it, involves embracing His miracle. One cannot ignore, merely tolerate, or simply just allow His miracle to come into life unnoticed or unappreciated. No, embracing His miracle involves receiving it eagerly and gladly; accepting it willingly.

What a blessing children are. For first time parents, as well as the seasoned parents, a new addition to the family is a celebration to anticipate. However, in our culture many continue pursuing the same life they had before children. Many view parenthood as beginning once the baby is born, not during pregnancy. Even though women today are told they are preparing by getting all the necessities in order, they still continue the same lifestyle and schedule up until the due date. Women struggle to adjust to their new role as mother as they deal with hormonal changes as well as the reality that their lives will never truly be the same. Men also have their ways of struggling to adjust to life with a new baby. Embracing the reality of parenthood can be very difficult for many, especially if their lifestyles reflected much independence. As Christians in today's culture, we need to adopt (another definition of embrace) a biblical perspective of parenthood, and intentionally prepare our lifestyles.

If you stop to think about the miracle of creation, it is awe-inspiring. God's miraculous handiwork is so intricate and unique. Marveling at His miraculous creation of your baby draws you into a deeper bond with your baby and your Lord. As you learn about how your baby is growing inside you and how your body was designed to nurture him/her, everything needed to grow deep within you, you will become more appreciative and amazed by your Creator. Surrendering any pride you may have taken in the creation of your baby and recognizing it was all God is the beginning of surrendering your child back to the Lord; which is something every parent needs to do in order for a healthy relationship to exist. One definition of embrace is "to take in with the eye or mind."[12] To study, learn, and/or understand the design and creation of your baby's body and soul in addition to the creation of your own and its ability to bring forth life is one way to embrace His miracle. Take in with your eyes and accept and believe with your mind the truth that is revealed through God's Word.

As Christians, we are so quick to take the glory for things that are God's. We need focus on giving Him all the glory for the great things He has done. The creation of your body, your baby, and all the miracles that surround birth are because of God's works, not ours. He designed your body as an intricate and beautiful system. Once you understand the purposes behind your body's responses, it is much easier to confidently embrace the reality of how birth works and surrender to the process without fear. He brings forth life and our lives are in His hands. To embrace His miracle, one has to acknowledge it is His miracle. We so quickly want and work hard at being in control of our lives, that it is not easy to embrace birth by letting Him have the control. In surrendering all to Jesus, you are in the safest hands, the hands of your Creator. In childbirth, we can plan and prepare until we are out of breath, but ultimately we need to give it back to God, letting Him reign in our lives. Embracing His headship over your birth requires embracing His headship over your life.

Another definition of embrace is "to avail oneself of: to embrace an opportunity." This new season or journey in one's life certainly does offer an opportunity for growth . . . and the key to experiencing that growth is embracing the journey. In childbirth, the pain of contractions indicates progress. It isn't a sign something is wrong, but rather a sign something is right. Do you remember getting growing pains when you were growing up? My children get them now and I find myself teaching them nothing is wrong, the growing pains mean they are growing. There are things you can do to relieve the pain, like massage, prayer, and even homeopathy, but the growing pains indicate you are growing!

Embracing the pain, the reality of parenthood, and that this miracle is God's and not all about you shows acceptance of this opportunity for growth. Embracing all of life's experiences, the blessings, the trials, and the sufferings in total surrender and trust is hard. In the midst of the pain, to choose to look for the good, choose to have a teachable heart and seek to grow through the experience is embracing life through a paradigm that is focused on God and His purposes.

Embracing your baby for the first time is filled with indescribable emotions and feelings. To put it simply—nothing else seems to matter in life at that very moment; you want to hold time still and just cuddle your blessing. Many describe the first few hours of embracing their children as life-changing experiences. I don't really think anything in life quite compares to it. When a woman deeply embraces God's miracle in her life and has been preparing her heart, home, soul, marriage, and life to receive this gift, the moment becomes even more spiritual. Her heart and soul are not distracted by anything or anyone. The more I focus on the Lord through my pregnancy and prepare my heart to receive more of Him and His blessings in my life, the more I value the gift, the more I treasure it and don't want to let it go.

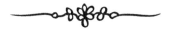

Prayer

Lord, I pray my sisters in the Lord who are reading this next section would embrace the truth about what You want to do in each of our lives through pregnancy, labor, birth, and motherhood. I pray that these words would be Your words, not my own. I thank You for what You have taught me Lord. Let it not be just for me but to encourage and uplift my sisters in the faith as they journey toward motherhood. May they be empowered and equipped with truth and understanding of what Your Word teaches. Thank You for this awesome privilege to learn more about You in my life and serve You in this way. May we all embrace Your miracles in our lives every day. May the words of my mouth and the meditations of my heart be pleasing to You, O God.

Beautiful Pain

No matter how you decide to birth your baby, medicated or not, all women experience some degree of pain in childbirth. The pain we experience is not often mentioned in a God glorifying way. My goal is that this chapter encourages all women, even those who decide not to have a natural birth. We can choose to cope with pain in a way that glorifies our Lord.

As we study the purpose behind the pain from both biblical and physiological perspectives, I pray you are empowered to embrace truth and the blessings to come. We also need to remember that only God is to be glorified, not the suffering or the pain, only Jesus.

Father,

You alone are worthy of glory. We are thankful for the ways you have created our bodies to deal with pain. We are also thankful for the advances you have allowed in the medical field, that we might receive assistance in emergencies. I pray as we look at pain and birth, that your truths would be revealed and empower my sisters who are seeking to have a deeper understanding of the purpose behind pain in childbirth. This is a tender subject Lord. Soften our hearts and help us to see you glorified. I pray that all of my sisters, regardless of how they experience birth, natural or not, would be encouraged in how You designed their bodies and that it would empower them to embrace more opportunities for growth in the future. Amen.

A Testimony of God's Grace and Redemption

The laboring became fast and furious. Never before had I been at a place where the pain was so overwhelming I could not speak. In my last birth experience I was able to exercise self-control over how much I focused on the pain. The Holy Spirit clearly had blessed me with the fruit of self-control over my emotions then, but why not now? I was struggling to focus. The contractions were literally right on top of each other, only three seconds apart. I could barely ask for prayer let alone worship with my lips; all of this lasted for about forty-five minutes. Though I could not sing with words man could hear, my spirit sang and lead me into true worship. My husband spoke confidence to me in a gentle whisper, "You were made to do this, remember." Yes, I do remember. At that moment I remembered our intimate conversation promptly after my first baby's birth. I had told him I felt like I was made to do this. Almost as quickly as I remembered saying those words, I regained confidence in the Lord to do this work again. That confidence empowered me to focus on the task at hand.

Just as I was nearing the end, I began fearing again. Then in my weakness, my midwife asked, "Do you feel the head crowning? Do you feel the ring of fire?" In that moment an image flashed in my mind of the crown of thorns that had been placed on the crown of my Savior's head. Easter had just passed a few weeks before and I vividly remembered the scene in *The Passion of the Christ* where they placed the crown of thorns on Jesus' head and He bled. As I remembered this, I cried, not in my pain, as much as in remembrance of my Savior's pain. I was distracted by the truth of how He bore my sins, and within in a few minutes I had my first-born son in my arms. The Lord delivered me again in that moment as I focused on Him. He delivered me and there was no more pain. Just as "a woman giving birth to a child has pain because her time has come; but when her baby is born she forgets the anguish because of her joy that a child is born into the world," (John 16:21 NIV).

When we focus on Him, He provides us those little whispers of truth that remind us of what He has done, and we forget about ourselves.

"Dear friends, do not be surprised at the painful trial you are suffering, as though something strange were happening to you. But rejoice in that you participate in the sufferings of Christ, so that you may be overjoyed when his glory is revealed."
1 Peter 4:12 (NIV)

Sisters, clearly birth is painful for most women. In my experiences there has always been an element of pain. Although for some, God may choose to deliver you from pain. We should be careful not to put God in a box so as to prevent us from crying out to Him for healing either for our sisters or ourselves. I do believe God has a purpose in allowing us to experience some pain, and my hope is in reflecting on the realities in our world today and studying God's purposes and His Word, you may be built up and encouraged, looking forward to engaging all He has for you in your personal experience.

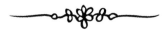

A Deeper Look at the False Teaching/Lie That Birth Is NOT Painful

Throughout history women have dreaded and feared birth because of the truth—childbirth is painful.

We have already discussed lies and fears women believe about birth as well as false teachings on the topic of pain in childbirth. If you were to search for a book on birth, you would find hundreds. Many are similar, in that they describe the stages of labor, how to cope with pain using different methodologies, and what to expect. All of this can prove to be very helpful, but there are deceptions within many spiritual and educational books on birth as well. These deceptions should be filtered through the word of God or Christians should guard their hearts from them entirely. For the Christian woman who wants to invite God into her experience, careful awareness is essential. We need to guard our minds against the new age or secular worldviews that taint our perspectives and expectations. We need to be careful not to group natural birth into a new age category, for doing such a thing would be like throwing the baby out with the bath water. Instead, we need to view natural birth as another opportunity for God to draw us to Himself, another avenue for Him to do a sanctifying work in our lives.

Beautiful as birth is, it is painful. Unfortunately, there are many professionals and experts who will advocate that it is not. Some even imply if you are experiencing pain, then you are not strong spiritually or have not prepared for birth. I am here, as an older woman who has birthed six children naturally, to tell you the simple truth: that birth has always been, still is, and will always be painful.

> *"As a woman with child and about to give birth writhes and cries out in her pain, so were we in your presence, O LORD." Isaiah 26:17, NIV*

> *"She was with child. She cried out in pain, laboring to give birth." Revelation 12:2*

> *"For we are God's masterpiece. He has created us anew in Christ Jesus, so that we can do the good things he has planned for us long ago." Ephesians 2:10, NLT*

For further study also see Isaiah 13:8; Isaiah 21:3; Micah 4:9; Psalm 48:6; Matthew 24:8.

The truth, as clearly stated in the Word of God, is that childbirth is going to be painful, but God will give us His grace. His grace can take many forms: experiencing His joy in the midst of pain, experiencing pleasure simultaneously with the pain, and some may experience His mercy and deliverance from pain entirely. God's plan for each of our unique experiences will be different, but glorious as He works all things together for the good of those who love Him.

As we continue to study pain and talk about pain and discover more of what scripture says, let's not forget God's sovereignty and grace which is free for all who believe in Him and call upon the name of Jesus. He is fully capable to do a powerful and mighty work of deliverance, but for some it may be deliverance from the pain and others it may be deliverance in and through the pain.

There are no scriptural references in the Old or New Testaments that indicate women will not experience some form of pain in childbirth. If that were so, why would the Lord choose to compare a woman's pain in birth to end times throughout Scripture? Jesus is teaching His disciples about end times. He warns them (and us),

> "Watch out that no one deceives you. Many will come in my name claiming, 'I am he.' And will deceive many. When you hear of wars and rumors of wars, do not be alarmed. Such things MUST happen, but the end [delivery/relief/salvation] is still to come. Nation will rise against nation, and kingdom against kingdom. There will be earthquakes in various places and famines. These are the beginning of birth pains. You must be on guard." (Mark 13:5-9, emphasis mine, also see: 2 Kings 18, 19)

Did you notice the word "must" in this passage? Such things must happen. Jesus was teaching end times would be painful, but the pain was necessary to be aware of the trials to come, to be on guard and alert.

God compares this Scripture to end times because He knew childbirth would always be painful, and therefore the Scriptures would always be relevant, further preserving its sufficiency. How pointless would those Scriptures be today if we had no pain in birth? Our understanding of these Scriptures is so much more rich and profound because we do still experience pain in birth. The truth we can rest in is not that of popular opinion, or what we want to believe or hear, but that of God's word. God has created us marvelously to do this good, hard work that he planned for us long ago (Eph.2:10).

Ladies, God warns all believers to be on guard. We need to be careful that what we read on the topic of childbirth is not feeding us an extra-biblical or secular worldview.

As childbearing women in the 21st century, we need to allow our minds to be transformed by the Word of God with regard to our views of pregnancy, childbirth, and motherhood. We have been deceived by our enemy to fear these experiences and transitions in life, as have the many generations before us. We need to have a healthy, balanced, and biblical view of childbirth with regard to fear, pain, emergencies, and the medical profession. We need to submit what we believe about birth under the headship of Christ.

In order to truly have a healthy perspective on birth, we need to do some study. When did women begin birthing babies in hospitals? Why?[13] We have tried to expose many of the lies taught today, but we all need to ask: what false teachings have led us astray? What does Scripture really say about birth and pain in birth?[*]

Now that we have thoroughly established that birth is and always will be painful from looking at Scripture, let's look at why it is such and discuss God's blessing in the pain.

---

[*] For a *Brief History on Childbirth* go to: http://redeemingchildbirth.com/ and search the free downloads.

Our Biblical Heritage & Generational Curse

In Genesis 2:15-17, we find the account of the order in which man was created and of his fellowship with God. After man was created God "took the man and put him in the garden to work it and keep it. And the Lord God commanded the man saying, 'You may surely eat of every tree of the garden, but of the tree of knowledge of good and evil you shall not eat, for in the day that you eat of it you shall surely die.'" God made this command clearly known to the man, before the woman was even created. God noticed there was a need to make a woman, a suitable helper. Out of His goodness and will to provide all the man needed, God caused Adam to fall into a deep sleep and took a rib with which He formed a woman. "Then the man said, 'This is bone of my bones and flesh of my flesh; she shall be called Woman, because she was taken out of man,'" (Gen. 3:23).

The First Discipline Man Experienced

Then came the temptation to sin. The woman clearly had been warned of the law to not eat of the tree of knowledge of good and evil that was in the garden; for when the serpent tempted her she knew it was against God's command. Still the serpent was crafty and convinced her to eat of the forbidden fruit. Following her transgression, she convinced her husband to also eat of the fruit, "She also gave some to her husband who was with her, and he ate," (Genesis 3:6).

Remember that the Lord had warned them they would surely die if they ate of the tree. To God's dismay and grief, His children disobeyed Him. After cursing the serpent, he disciplined the woman and the man. To the woman (who still had no other name), He said, "I will surely multiply your pain in childbearing; in pain you shall bring forth children. Your desire shall be for your husband, and he shall rule over you." To Adam he said, "Because you have listened to the voice of your wife and have eaten of the tree of which I commanded you, 'You shall not eat of it,' cursed is the ground because of you; in pain you shall eat of it all the days of your life; thorns and thistles shall it bring forth for you and you shall eat of the plants of the field. By the sweat of your face you shall eat bread, till you return to the ground for out of it you were taken; for you are dust and to dust you shall return," (Gen. 3:16-19).

God's discipline for this original sin was given to all men and women. But pain in childbirth is not the generational "curse." God did not give us pain in birth as our "punishment." As we discuss in the next chapter "Understanding God's Design," God created Eve's body the same as He created ours. He created our body to have contractions to help ad us in bringing forth life. The consequence for original sin is sharpened pain, greatly increased pain, multiplied pain, or multiplied sorrow, not pain in general. Nowhere in scripture does it indicate that Eve would have had a pain-free birth before the fall. We do know that after He created Eve, with her ability to bring forth life, He saw that His work was complete and good.

The generational curse that we struggle with is not that birth is painful. In fact I don't even like calling it a curse. The only thing "generational" we struggle with is our sin and desire to blame others for what we experience. It is that because of our sin, we experience separation from God and we often focus on ourselves and not on God's purposes or plan. Just as sin is a generational sin, for women multiplied pains in birth is generational. But our sin wants to call pain a curse or a burden. In the next chapter we discuss God's design and how our pain is actually a physiological trigger for helping us cope with the pain. When we focus on the why behind the pain and we allow it to just be and engage it with God's help, rather than avoiding it, and we understand the greater purposes behind the pain, it somehow can make it all worth it, beautiful.

God's discipline for this original sin was given to us all, men and women. God clearly spoke to Adam and Eve as a Father in remorse for His precious children's ill decision, for they had sinned for the first time.

The punishment was a direct consequential discipline for the original sin; both Adam and Eve were punished in direct correlation to their primary purposes and the original will of God.

Then when God disciplined mankind after the fall, He chose not to remove that original blessing of procreation "to be fruitful and multiply" (Gen. 3:28) even though they had just committed original sin. Eve would be blessed to bring forth life even though she herself would experience multiplied pain in childbearing. For now, they were allowed to live and experience the joy of having children. Yes they would die eventually, but Adam chose to focus on the good and name her "mother of all the living." We, too, have the choice, to look at the good. Though we will have pain in childbirth, as one of my midwives put it, we can be thankful for every strong contraction because it causes progress toward having the baby delivered. As the author Gills wrote about Eve, "In sorrow shall thou bring forth children, sons and daughters, with many severe pangs and sharp pains, which are so very acute, that great tribulations and afflictions are often in Scripture set forth by them: and it is remarked by naturalists, that women bring forth their young with more pain than any other creature."[14] We can learn from Adam's example, to look for the good and have gratitude.

Just as the Word says, we will surely die and thorns and thistles do still grow in our gardens and fields of wheat. We still experience pain in childbearing. Though not every man may physically work a field or farm, he is called to work hard and not to be lazy. The prosperity of our country has made life easier in many regards, so much so that an entitlement attitude has infiltrated our society. Many do not have the desire to work hard or the perspective that one reason for their creation was for work. As our culture grows farther from that truth we grow more entitled. For many, that entitlement attitude leads to the belief that they do not deserve to experience any pain. The medical industry further exacerbates the problem by offering medications like candy. Both men and women today need to focus on reclaiming the curse of hard work and walking through trials and pain, for in doing so is a great reward. The reward is knowing God in a new way that comes only from being empty and experiencing His strength to accomplish a task.

So why would any woman want to choose natural birth, knowing full well it will be painful when she can simply opt out?

Knowing God intimately as Deliverer comes from experiencing Him deliver you from pain, suffering, or mourning. Unfortunately, one cannot experience Him as the Deliverer if they do not undergo pain or suffering. Because we are all sinners and have much to be saved from, for those who have received the Lord and surrendered their lives under His headship, we can find unity in all knowing Him as our Savior. In childbirth we simply have another opportunity, as in undergoing other pains in life as well, to surrender and experience Him faithfully and mercifully as our Deliverer. None of us will truly know, until the day of our reunion in heaven with our Lord, quite what it means to be Delivered, but we can grow in our faith in Him and in the hope of what is to come as we experience His graces in this life, walking with us through pain. We have many opportunities for experiencing God as the deliverer in this fallen life. Natural childbirth is simply an opportunity to know God better through another experience. In birth we are once again in a position of needing our Savior, and this journey of experiencing Him rescue us and bless us can impress upon our hearts and souls a deeper understanding of the grace He has given us.

Nowhere in the Old or New Testaments does God promise this life will be pain free if we believe in Him. In fact, it is all quite the contrary. He warns us of the days to come. We should expect persecution, pain, suffering, agony, and more while here on earth. We are to yearn for our heavenly home; it is there we will not experience pain. The power of the cross for today lies in our relationship with Him and our capacity to give up control to Him, allowing Him to do His will in our lives. Romans 8:18 reveals there are present sufferings and that these will be sanctifying, "I consider that our present sufferings are not worth comparing with the glory that will be revealed in us." The growth that takes place will create a glory revealed within us.

We are still subject to the adversities of this life that exist because of sin. We live in a sinful world; that is our reality. The consequence of sin is death. When we sin, others are affected by our sin. When others sin, we are affected by their sin. The punishment from the fall was death. We all die, that is our reality. Jesus was our perfect example of how to glorify God through surrender to His will while emotionally suffering (see Jesus' prayer in the Garden of Gethsemane, Matthew 26:36-43). He showed us how to gracefully submit to whatever pain the Lord allows, trusting the Father knows best. Jesus taught us how to lay down our personal preferences, our personal opinions, and our crosses in order to take up His. In physical suffering and pain, Jesus showed us how to die to ourselves, fully surrendered into the hands of the Father. "To this you were called, because Christ suffered for you, leaving you an example, that you should follow in his steps," (1 Peter 2:21). Just as we cannot escape death, which was part of the punishment for eating the fruit of the tree; likewise we all still have to live with the consequences of original sin. Weeds and thistles still grow, and women still experience pain and sorrow in childbirth.

God is your Father in heaven, who loves you deeply and wants you to hear His voice and know Him intimately. If you look at the Christian life, one could agree most are drawn to the Lord in times of trial, suffering, and pain. I believe God wants that from all of us, all the time. Not just in times of need. He wants you to draw near to Him. Though pain in childbirth is not ideal, most of us would agree if there were no pain in childbirth it would be a much more desirable life event. As Christians we remember the promises of God in His Word. Knowing the blessing from that comes in having children, an eternal relationship with them, inspires us to have children regardless of the potential pain and trials down the road. Just as we have an eternal perspective on the lives of our children, we should also have an eternal perspective on the spiritual growth caused by persevering through the pain. Because of the pain experienced in birth, couples are much more thankful for the birth of a healthy child and the preservation of a healthy mother. If it were easy, I do believe that sadly, our hearts would grow colder toward recognizing God's blessings in these circumstances. We would begin to exhibit an entitlement attitude of expecting easy births and healthy babies, rather than having a heart of gratitude toward God when we do.

The Curse and the Cross

I have heard of women believing before birth, "I don't have to experience any pain in childbirth, Jesus died for my sin and for the curse." Unfortunately, many women are extremely discouraged during childbirth when they find they are experiencing immense pain. The unfortunate fact is that this statement or belief is somewhat extra-biblical. There are many New Testament scriptures that describe women experiencing pain in childbirth, before and after the life, death and resurrection of Christ. "For when they are saying, 'Peace and safety,' then sudden destruction will come on them, like birth pains on a pregnant woman; and they will in no way escape," (1 Thess. 5:3). The apostles themselves use women experiencing pain in childbirth as an analogy to make points throughout the Scriptures.

Since we are all born into original sin, we all experience the generational consequence (punishment) of that original sin. Jesus came and died for all our sins, including original sin, that we might have eternal life. He came to give us freedom from our eternal fate if we receive His free gift of salvation. The reality of God's punishment for this original sin is that it still stands, just as we still struggle with our original sinful nature. However, living in the power of the Holy Spirit we can have victories over our sins as we choose in every moment whether to lean on Him for strength in the good fight against our flesh. In childbirth, we women can have victory as well when we choose to give glory to God, even in the pain. Not allowing the pain or fear to dictate our ability to let His Spirit (dwelling within us) have authority over our minds, emotions, and physical bodies gives us victory over our selfish nature. Jesus dying for our sins doesn't mean we won't experience pain on earth, it means we will have Him to walk through it with us, equipping us to endure, and to do it well.

The Lord longs to be gracious to you, to show you mercy and grace. He longs to be intimate with you. He has provided you with an opportunity to grow in Him. Embrace and use this time while you are pregnant to really grow in the Lord. Allow the Lord to use this life transition to do what he has intended to do; to prepare you for motherhood. I am so thankful I have forty weeks to work at preparing my heart through submission to my Lord, to welcome a new family member.

> *"Yet the Lord longs to be gracious to you; he rises to show you compassion. For the Lord is a God of Justice. Blessed are all who wait for him!"*
> Isaiah 30:18

In our finite minds we cannot see our futures; we cannot see any good that could come from the suffering or pain we are enduring in the moment. It is our nature to become focused inward rather than upward. Childbirth is painful, but the pain lasts a short time and the beauty lasts forever. In the pain of childbirth, there are many blessings to be experienced. It is the most rewarding pain you will ever experience in your life: one with no regrets, one that comes with an eternal blessing.

If we can focus upward to God, and see the good in the outcome of the process of birth, we can endure and experience joy and thanksgiving in the midst of pain. The precious gift of a child is worth all the pain. When one chooses to focus on this blessing, the process by which the baby is born becomes beautiful. The love of a mother to give birth and not give up becomes beautiful to witness and experience. The pain is a beautiful description of a mother's love.

In childbirth, pain is an indicator of growth. At the first indication of a contraction or back pain, a woman knows her laboring is progressing. We have an opportunity for many kinds of growth in life. We have the opportunity to grow in any trials we experience. If we seek God and lean on Him, persevering and staying faithful in our belief in Him and His goodness, we will be blessed with all kinds of spiritual growth. Unfortunately, because our culture has compartmentalized pregnancy and birth to the medical professionals, we do not seek spiritual advice as often with regard to preparing for this life-changing event.

When you are in the midst of labor and delivery, you can choose which perspective of pain you want to embrace. You can both focus on the pain and dwell on it, growing weary in your own strength, or you can view the pain as progress and as an opportunity to grow in your relationship with the Lord and even those laboring with you. The pain becomes beautiful once you embrace the perspective of the potential outcome; the beauty that is going to be developed in your spiritual walk with the Lord. As God blesses you with what you need to endure, you will discover attributes of God that maybe you didn't know personally before, deepening your relationship with Him. As you pursue intimacy with Christ by leaning on Him, crying out to Him, worshiping Him, praying to Him with your husband because you truly, sincerely, NEED God in that moment, you are beautiful.

Embrace God's plan for your life as a woman and mother. You were created for such a time as this. He has full confidence in His design and He longs for you to rely on Him and grow in Him.

Every aspect of pregnancy and birth can be a blessing. It's all in how we choose to look at it. After all, it was the first blessing God gave to mankind, to be fruitful and multiply.

A critical note from the author on pain, suffering, sanctification, and glorifying God:

Before ending this chapter on pain, I feel compelled to share with you my heart. I do not in any way want anyone to read this chapter on pain in childbirth or the chapter titled "1 Timothy 2:15" which talks about birth as a sanctifying and spiritually growing experience and mistake the intent of the message. We are not to pursue injury or harm to our babies or ourselves. We are not to glorify suffering and walk around arrogantly flaunting how we conquered over it (when in reality it was not because of ourselves anyway).

As Christians, we need to be very careful not to glorify anything or anyone above God. As we strive to glorify Him in our life experiences, good and bad, we need to be on guard not to glorify the suffering or the blessing, but rather magnify His name and give Him the glory He alone deserves, as He enriches us through those painful experiences. It is His ability, not ours, to bring beauty out of our struggles. When we shine in our weakness, it isn't us shining; it is the Holy Spirit shining His light through us.

Childbirth is inevitably and predictably painful, even if for a short time. Do we turn in fear? No, but neither should we approach pain or walk away from birth thinking more highly of ourselves than we ought. Instead, our focus needs to be on glorifying our Lord and Savior. We need to make the choices He has given us freedom to make, in obedience to His personal call on our lives. We need to be careful not to make an idol out of natural childbirth or being strong enough to endure the pain, but rather only seek to praise Him, glorify Him, magnify Him, and allow the work of the Holy Spirit to be done in our lives and those who witness our births. Our lives are not just about us, they are about Him.

May I Pray for You?

Lord Jesus, we praise You that we are fearfully and wonderfully made. We are in awe that You would choose to bless us with the ability to bring forth life. What an incredible privilege it is to serve You and to be chosen by You to be the earthly mothers of these sweet children. I thank You for my sisters who are reading this book, Lord. May You speak to their hearts and souls. Reveal yourself to them in a new way. May your relationship with each of them be strengthened as they pursue to invite you into this intimate experience. I pray Lord, that as they prepare their birth plans that they would be wise, filtering all things through your Word. I pray they would seek Your will for their lives and this experience. I pray for you to bring a few special friends into their lives who can encourage, equip, and empower them toward following Your heart and embracing all life offers. Lord, help all of us to be strong women who live what we believe. I pray Lord that we would come humbly before you now, willing to let you refine our hearts. Help us all to trust you more Lord.

May we all be women who humbly submit to your headship and willingly take up Your cross. May we seek you in all things, including birth. Lord speak to my sisters. May they be encouraged this day to come before you with humble hearts, willing to work with you toward spiritual growth through childbirth. Lord, you are our Deliverer, our Savior, and our Creator. Just as you delivered your people out of hardships all throughout Scripture, and you helped Eve bring forth man, Lord I ask you to do the same in my sisters' lives. Show them your goodness. Lord, bless them. Revive our hearts again. Let us see your glory Lord! Thank you Lord for the blessings you have given us already. We remember what you have done in our lives. Thank you Lord for your promises, for they are new every morning and your word endures forever. May your

Kingdom come. May your will be done, on earth as it is in heaven. Lord, bless us so we can be a blessing to others and share of Your mighty works in our lives. Thank you for the children you are blessing us with Lord; please prepare us to be all they need us to be. Walk with us, continue to refine us and teach us. Help us to serve our families with loving and grateful hearts unto you. Thank you for giving us this opportunity for growth. We love you Lord Jesus. Amen.

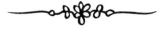

Understanding God's Design

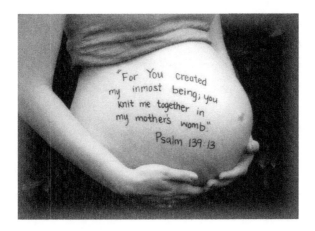

"For You created my inmost being; you knit me together in my mother's womb."
Psalm 139:13

Recognizing His Design:
He Prepared Our Bodies for Birth

Take faith sister, God has designed your body for childbirth. Having confidence and faith God designed your body to do this sanctifying work is part of the process by which He is redeeming childbirth. Reconciling our perspectives on pain and how He created us to the truths found in His Word redeems something that has been lost, or forgotten.

God created us with the amazing mechanics to give birth. He created the birth process. What He created is good. The curse of pain was also meant for our good, not only to bring us into deeper fellowship with our

Creator, but also to trigger pain warriors built within our bodies. God created our bodies with a natural response to pain called beta-endorphins.

Endorphins are only created and released when our nervous system indicates pain. God gave these natural endorphins to us, because He is so good and He never gives us more than we can handle.

> "Our bodies produce brain chemicals called endorphins in response to pain or stress. When mothers get epidural anesthesia for childbirth they don't produce those pain-relieving endorphins. We know that maternal endorphins readily cross the placenta and affect the baby. Endorphins travel to our babies as well and if medication is administered to the mother, her body will not create the natural endorphins, which means the baby won't get this natural pain killer either." Carol Gray, Midwife, Infant Craniosacral Therapist

Endorphins are one of the blessings that God has given us so our bodies can physically cope with the pain of childbirth, but they only work if you do not confuse them. Have confidence in God the Creator who made your body specifically for birthing and believe in His ability to give you the supernatural strength, to both endure the pain and thrive spiritually while embracing the pain. He set us up for success by creating our bodies with the right neurological response patterns, hormones, and natural painkillers. We are so blessed to have the knowledge of how God designed our bodies to give birth and how we have everything we need to do it well.

To further encourage your faith in His creation of beautiful you, here are other effects of beta-endorphins:[15]

- Beta-endorphins are a naturally occurring opiates that act to restore homeostasis (internal balance) in the body. They are secreted by the pituitary gland in times of pain and stress.

- Studies suggest that beta-endorphins increase tolerance to pain and suppress the immune system, both of which are important during birth.

- Beta-endorphins promote the release of prolactin during labor, which prepares the mother's breasts for lactation and aids in lung maturation for the baby.

The Influence Interventions Have on Beta-Endorphins

It has been scientifically proven through testing and documented that epidurals affect a woman's natural hormones, which, in turn, can interfere, reduce, and inhibit beta-endorphins.

According to Dr. Sarah Buckley, "Beta-endorphin also switches on learning and memory, perhaps explaining why we remember our labor and birth in such amazing detail."[16] So if we are switching off these natural brain chemicals unnecessarily . . . well you do the math! Does it make any mathematical sense to prevent all of the benefits above that come from the release of beta-endorphins in exchange for pain abatement?

Other Blessings God Created Us with

God not only blessed us with beta-endorphins, but also with hormones such as estrogen and progesterone, oxytocin, prolactin, and catecholamines (epinephrine/adrenaline and norepinephrine/ noradrenaline).

Dr. Sarah Buckley writes:

"Oxytocin plays several important roles after birth. High levels of oxytocin produced as the baby stimulates the mother's breast help keep the uterus contracted and prevent postpartum hemorrhage. Oxytocin mediates the 'milk ejection reflex' which allows for successful breastfeeding.

And, as the hormone of love, oxytocin promotes the development of a strong bond between mother and baby.

Oxytocin has another crucial role to play after birth. Oxytocin causes the contractions that lead to separation of the placenta from the uterus, and its release as the 'after-birth.' When oxytocin levels are high, strong contractions occur that reduce the chance of bleeding or post-partum hemorrhage.

"There are more than three hundred known bodily effects of prolactin, including induction of maternal behavior, increase in appetite and food intake, suppression of fertility, stimulation of motor and grooming activity, reduction of the stress response, stimulation of oxytocin secretion and opiod activity, alteration of the sleep-wake cycle and increase in REM sleep, reduction of body temperature, and pain relief. Prolactin, along with growth hormone, is one of the hormones of growth and lactation and as such has a crucial influence in the development and function of the immune system."[17]

Prolactin is best known for its benefits after birth, especially with breast-feeding, bonding, and emotions. Combined with oxytocin, the two are a strong duo of emotional support and balance for the new mother as she bonds with and nurtures her baby. Unfortunately, these hormones and painkillers only act at their most optimal levels when *uninhibited by synthetic drugs.* The moment that synthetic drugs are used most all of these hormonal benefits are prevented.

I am clearly not covering all the awesome details of how God has blessed us by creating our bodies ready for childbirth. This is just a glimpse of His creation. We can find confidence in the truth that God created our bodies to birth babies. He set up all the mechanics to work together. One of my dear midwives taught me while I was laboring to focus on how each contraction and pain was a gift, making progress toward the moment when I would have my baby in my arms.

When we focus on the good and the blessings, our focus is no longer on getting rid of the pain, but rather on embracing it and letting it take its course within our bodies. We can trust that the God, who created us in our mothers' wombs and brought us forth, is the same designer.

Choosing to focus on the heavenly things, on Jesus, takes strength and intentionality. Remembering the blessings He has created within your body is encouraging and empowering regardless of the way you give birth (natural or not).

My prayer is that this particular chapter has equipped some of you with deeper convictions as to why you can trust God's design of your body to bring forth life.

May you focus on Him, and believe that birth cannot only be manageable but a wonderful and spirit-building experience. I often describe my birth experiences as painful yet sustained by the Spirit of the living God, feeling His presence and strengthened by Him to accomplish the task set before me. By the design and strength of the Lord, I have brought forth six babies into this world. It was not by my own power, but by Jesus and His power to save and deliver. He truly delivered my babies, in His timing. He held my babies in his hands the whole time, just as He did while they were in my womb, being created by Him, and protected by Him. Jesus is creating and preparing you and your baby in much the same way right now.

1 Timothy 2:15

Saved through childbearing? At first glance, this verse can seem very confusing.

Yet she will be saved in childbearing. Saved. What does that mean? At first glance, I have to admit, I found myself baffled by the true meaning behind this verse. After much researching, I found the answer to be very simple. Simple as it may be—it's easy to say, but hard to do. Isn't that how life is with regard to surrendering our will under the headship of our Lord? It may seem a simple concept to understand, but actually taking action on it is sometimes a harder. The meaning behind this scripture passage is not an easy one to preach today. This Scripture has been mistakenly explained to mean that woman earn salvation through giving birth. We are NOT saved by our works; therefore we cannot earn our salvation by giving birth (see Galatians 5:1-8). This particular verse, 1 Timothy 2:15, was meant to be understood in conjunction with the fullness of salvation as recorded in the Word of God.

> *"Yet she will be saved through childbearing—if they continue in faith and love and holiness, with self-control."*
> 1 Timothy 2:15

Sisters, let me begin this section by saying if you do not understand any of the terms mentioned in this chapter, go to your husband, and/or your pastor to help you see the full meaning of the gift of salvation and redemption by studying it. I am not going to be able to cover all that is implied in this passage in this one chapter. However, I eagerly encourage you to engage in studying these "Christian-ese" (Christian- specific) terms. They are truly foundational to the depth of our understanding the fullness of what Christ died for. I have personally experienced an enriched devotion time with the Lord having done all of the research for this chapter and pray that you would be inspired to act with a similar hunger for truth and knowledge. Ladies, I am an ordinary stay-at-home mama of six very busy young children. I know how hard it is to find time to invest in studies for yourself when you are constantly focused on the studies of your children, believe me. But we have an extraordinary God, a gentle Shepherd who wants us to yearn for Him. Let the Lord guide you as you seek Him. He wants to give you His wisdom and understanding and open your eyes to the empowering truths in His Word.

So as you read through the thoughts on 1 Timothy 2:15 in this chapter, jot down words that seem unfamiliar and go look them up. Look up the verses mentioned in this chapter and cross-reference the verses, I promise you will be blessed.

So let's dig in; clearly, **we are not saved by childbearing in the sense of earning our salvation, so what does it mean?** As I mentioned before, to understand this verse one needs to understand the fullness of what comprises salvation.

Jesus died for our sins so that we might be redeemed and so we might live a redeemed life here on earth.

> "He who supposes that Jesus Christ only lived and died again in order to provide justification and forgiveness of sins for His people has yet much to learn. Whether he knows it or not, he is dishonoring our blessed Lord, and making Him only half a Savior. The Lord has undertaken everything that His people's should require; not only to deliver them from the guilt of their sins by His atoning death, but from dominion of their sins, by placing in their hearts the Holy Spirit; not only to justify them, but also to sanctify them (1 Cor.1:30)," by J.C. Ryle[18]

As Christians, we can live in freedom from the spiritual bondage of an eternal death because Jesus has justified us, giving us the free gift of eternal life. Jesus died so we could have eternal life. He did the work; we cannot do anything to deserve this grace. We are justified and redeemed. He also died so we could live in freedom from the bondage of sin while here on earth. This is done through the process of sanctification. Justification is a gift; sanctification is a process every believer has to experience personally. Sanctification is the aspect of the pilgrim's progress that requires surrender. We know that because we have been forgiven. We can experience living with love, joy, peace, and grace but it is the Holy Spirit who creates the hunger for living in righteousness and pursuing growth. It is living all of life on purpose that is the result of a journey of surrendering to sanctification.

> *"He Himself bore our sins in His body on the tree, that we might die to sin and live to righteousness. By his wounds you have been healed."*
> *1 Peter 2:24*

Brief explanation of the difference between justification and sanctification

Jesus died for our sin, so that we may be redeemed, born again, through justification and sanctification. Justification is something only Jesus can do; we cannot justify ourselves through any means of works. His work on the cross justified us. Jesus has redeemed us, being the one true atoning sacrifice. Justification is the gift of being forgiven, justified, and given the gift of eternal life.

Sanctification is the refining process of being conformed more and more to the image of God—what God wants us to be. It is the process we live everyday as we run the race striving to live righteously, glorifying the Lord. Sanctification is a co-dependent process, a partnership in which by **the prompting of the Holy Spirit**, we surrender to the refining; correction, pain, and suffering the Lord may use to grow us (sanctify us). Remember that because it requires the prompting of the Holy Spirit, it is still God's doing in our life and not our own. The Holy Spirit who dwells within us leads us to full surrender to the Lord and His purposes.

Sanctification Is Growth

"Regeneration is birth; sanctification is growth. In regeneration God implants desires that were not there before: desire for God, for holiness, and for hallowing and glorifying God's name in this world; desire to pray, worship, love, serve, honor, and please God; desire to show love and bring benefit to other. Regeneration is a momentary monergistic act of quickening the spiritually dead. As such it was God's work alone. Sanctification, however, is in one synergistic—it is an ongoing cooperative process in which regenerate persons, alive to God and freed to sin's dominion (Rom. 6:11, 14-18), are required to exert themselves in sustained obedience. God's method of sanctification is neither activism (self-reliant activity) nor apathy (God reliant passivity), but God-dependent effort (2 Cor.7: 1; Phil.3: 10-14; Heb. 12:14). Knowing that without Christ's enabling, we can do nothing, morally speaking, as we should, and that he is ready to strengthen us for all that we have to do (Phil.4: 13)." J.I. Packer[19]

Sanctification is the process the Christian undergoes in this life. It is the process by which Jesus refines us and makes us more holy. As we are transformed by the power of His spirit in our lives, we can become more like Him and have victory over our sins. Because of Him, we can obey and have self-control, as well as all other gifts of the Spirit. We need to become imitators of Christ, so as to "let your light shine before others, so that they may see your good works and give glory to your Father who is in heaven," (Matt. 5:16). We need to be transformed more into His likeness from our sinful nature to be able to desire the things God Himself desires. For our hearts to become more like our Father's so we might obey and "Therefore go and make disciples of all nations, baptizing them in the name of the Father and of the Son and of the Holy Spirit," (Matt. 28:19). Being focused on Jesus while in childbirth, surrendered to the Holy Spirit, empowers you to become an imitator of Christ in pain, willingly accepting the pain in the moment for the blessing in the end. Being focused on Jesus enables you to think bigger than yourself, being sensitive to ministering to those around you, witnessing to nurses, doctors, midwives, and family members. It is hard to focus on these things in the midst of having contractions, but when we pursue God's purposes for our births and look to serve Him in it, He provides the strength and the focus of mind so He may be glorified.

Sanctification is the component of salvation referred to in 1 Timothy 2:15.

It makes perfect sense that sanctification occurs as a part of the salvation process. Sanctification is a work not often mentioned with regard to childbirth. Although by its definition, any woman who has had an aided or natural birth would agree that it is a sanctifying experience.

The Holy Spirit is doing a sanctifying work in a woman's heart and soul through child bearing, preparing her for the nurturing and selfless journey of motherhood.

It is so beautiful that the Lord provided women this universal opportunity for growth, which is usually in an earlier season in a woman's life. I believe this is strategically placed in our lives to prepare us for what is ahead in the life-long labor of motherhood. Every life experience leaves its mark on us, and if we engage them as opportunities for sanctification or growth in our relationship with the Lord, we will be on the path of living a life of "faith, love and holiness, with self-control." (1 Tim. 2:15)

Childbirth better prepares parents for the unending labor of love of parenthood. When a woman experiences the presence of the Lord in such an intimate way in her birth, she is equipped with a stronger faith, which in turn empowers her to gracefully do the hard work raising ambassadors for Christ. All of these attributes are greatly needed for motherhood. Being a parent reveals our own selfishness at times, and it isn't pretty. Parenthood is sanctifying in its own right. Our sin is ugly, but the beauty is found in the result of the sanctifying experience, which leads to spiritual maturity, humility, forgiveness, grace, and freedom from the bondage of sin while we live here on this earth. One cannot ever truly be ready for parenthood, but embracing the journey God has laid out for you in getting there is part of His way of preparing you. It is not easy, but neither is parenthood. I believe every part of the journey, when fully embraced, plays a part in the preparation.

Every opportunity to surrender our lives and hardships under Jesus' headship is an opportunity for growth in our relationship with Him. Every time we exercise our faith through the actions of obedience in trust, surrendering our lives gets a little easier. As Christians, we need to choose to create a habit out of everyday obedience to Christ. These are examples of how sanctification is truly a partnership, whereby we actively choose to walk through the situation, crisis, or experience and look for what God wants to teach us in it. When a woman chooses to trust God, and not fear, and experiences the Lord providing for her needs in birth so that she can endure, it builds her confidence in His faithfulness, strength and presence in her life. That trust is a precious asset to cling to throughout life. As one ages, we deal with all kinds of sufferings: disease, accidents, and death. As Christians, we are warned and encouraged to be prepared mentally for trials, to expect persecution for our faith. "Dear friends, **do not be surprised at the painful trial you are suffering,** as though something strange were happening to you. **But rejoice** that you participate in the sufferings of Christ, so that you may be overjoyed when his glory is revealed," (1 Peter 4:12,13, NIV, emphasis mine). We should not expect life to be easy or try to avoid it when it is hard, but instead look at the opportunity to learn more about God, more about what Jesus endured for us. When we experience trials and pain, it will create in us a yearning for our heavenly home.

Sanctification in Pregnancy & Childbirth

During pregnancy, we have a little accountability partner who walks with us, lies with us, and is with us, and in us all the time—our babies we carry in our wombs. When I am pregnant, I am constantly aware my baby is hearing my voice and being feeling my emotions. I am already parenting as a pregnant woman. If we as mothers and wives, for example, do not exercise self-control over our tongues or our anger, we are already molding our children's impressions of us in regard to how we handle conflict and how we react to circumstances. As I am raising other children, I think to myself: "Be careful Angie, do not loose self-control. You could frighten your baby by yelling." We need to recognize we have a very real accountability partner with us, in us, all the time. 1 Cor. 6:19 asks, "Do you not know that your body is a temple of the Holy Spirit, who is in you, whom you have received from God?" Pregnancy is a good training ground for submitting our emotions unto the Lord and practicing self-control.

For those who experience difficult pregnancies (morning sickness, bed rest, etc.), there are many opportunities for sanctification and refinement. See the chapter titled "Kneeling at the Porcelain Throne."

Pregnancy can be a sacrifice of sorts. If you are one to get morning sickness during pregnancy, then you know of the refining process that one grows through, especially in regard to having more children. For some, physically difficult pregnancies make the decision to surrender to another nine months of sickness, in order to receive another blessing from the Lord a harder decision. It is ugly looking at our self-preserving thoughts and motives sometimes; it is refining to look in that mirror.

As the expecting day grows closer and closer, the temptation to become anxious rather than patient grows harder and harder. The anticipation builds up as the expectant parents await the day they will hold their baby in their arms. If the woman goes overdue, it can become even harder to wait patiently and contentedly. This training in patience and trust in the Lord is another sanctifying aspect of pregnancy. Good training for parenthood.

In labor, a woman is challenged in so many countless ways:

- To surrender to the pain and allow it to take it's course in the process.

- To be light-hearted and thankful for each contraction, knowing each hard contraction is bringing her closer to holding her baby and being delivered from the pain.
- To have faith God is in control, leaning on Him, relying on His strength to endure.
- To take thoughts captive and choosing to think on those things that are praise worthy rather than allowing our fears to overwhelm us and make us tense.
- To trust in God's design of our bodies to do this good work.

Most women are in immense pain during childbirth. When any person is in physical pain, her true nature toward God is revealed. She is either cursing Him, praising Him, ignoring Him, or trying to take control herself. It is easy to praise Him in good times, but very hard to glorify Him in suffering, no matter what the case of suffering. This is a sanctifying experience, because our pure nature is revealed: one of surrender to fear or strength in the Lord, one of anger and lack of self-control of the tongue, or one of a gentle and peace-filled spirit. The fruit of the Spirit is either displayed or not.

There is a continued opportunity for sanctification after birth, to remain humble, not thinking too highly of ourselves and to "continue in faith and love and holiness, with self-control," (1 Tim. 2:15).

Our reliance on Christ can be portrayed in our births if we purpose to involve Him. What a challenge, to remain in Him while in such pain. Experiencing labor with the help of the Lord is a milestone in life. When you rely on Him for strength through trust and He provides, your faith is multiplied. When the Lord multiplies your faith, it better prepares you for those circumstances in life you will encounter, experiences that require immense faith and trust.

Since sanctification is a partnership, a co-dependent work, our responsibility is in choosing to embrace the experiencing God allows in our lives to grow us and then we seek to look for the lesson, the reason, the why, because that is where the spiritual growth takes place.

We are to submit and surrender to the Lord completely in every area of our lives. This is a conviction we hold that has been revealed to us through the truth we have chosen to believe in the Word of God. Surrendering all includes allowing the Lord to do a sanctifying work in us, through our everyday lives, trials, sufferings, and even through our pain in childbearing. We grow closer to Christ as we surrender more of our lives, even by submitting our childbirth unto Him. To submit is a choice. A choice we have to proactively surrender to. It requires acknowledging in the moment of pain, trial, or suffering that this is a time where God could make us more holy, if we let Him. Letting Him sanctify us by growing our relationship with Him through prayer, reliance upon Him, through praising and worshipping Him in our pain, we will grow. When we go through any situation or trail in life we are faced with a choice—to let it get us down and surrender to it, or to surrender it unto the Lord and let Him redeem it by doing a sanctifying (growing) work in us. It is a choice.

"And because of him you are in Christ Jesus, who became to us righteousness and sanctification and redemption, so that, as it is written, 'Let one who boasts, boast in the Lord.'"
1 Corinthians 1:30-31

Pray with me

Father God, thank you for sending your one and only Son to redeem us, cleanse us, forgive us, and make it possible for us to enter into your presence. Thank you especially for the gift of eternal life, where we will no longer labor and struggle to surrender all to You. Thank you for not leaving us alone but providing us with a wise Counselor to guide us while we discern how to best follow you. Lord, pregnancy, labor, and birth are sanctifying, but so are motherhood and life in general. Please give us grace to live our lives in full surrender and willing to open our hearts to the opportunities of growth You have planned for us. May they not be wasted, but utilized for the advancement of your Kingdom. Amen.

Fruitful Surrender

Preparing Your Heart for the Sanctifying Work in Birth

"Trust in him at all times, O people; pour out your hearts to him, for God is our refuge. Selah"
Psalm 62:8

Can any of us really be prepared for Christ to do a sanctifying work in us? Are we ever prepared for God to grow us, to sanctify us through any struggle, fear, pain, or life transition?

I remember as a child always wanting to be older, bigger, so I could have more responsibility. I think most children have that insatiable desire to grow. To be big. Never fully satisfied with simply being children. The reality though is that with physical or emotional growth, often there are growth pains. So is the case

"He put a new song in my mouth, a hymn of praise to our God. Many will see and fear and put their trust in the LORD. Blessed is the man who makes the LORD his trust, who does not look to the proud, to those who turn aside to false gods"
Psalm 40:3,4 (NIV)

with the growth that comes through sanctification. Though the outcome is always worth it, the growth process itself is sometimes painful.

We understand physical growth pains are a normal part of physical growth, trusting that the pain is a sign that growth is happening. So it is with spiritual growth. As women who have been gifted the privilege to bring forth life, we need to

anticipate God's sanctifying growth. But we have a choice in how we view that growth. As I experienced contractions in labor, I called them "good ones." Each contraction growing more intense meant I was that much closer to meeting my baby, face to face. The Holy Spirit transformed my perspective of the contractions into what they were in light of God's perfect design, a gift, as painful as they were.

Contractions are a part of God's perfect design. They were not the curse. Before God greatly increased pain in childbirth, He designed our bodies as He designed Eve's, including contractions, and they were good.

> *"This I declare about the LORD: He alone is my refuge, my place of safety; he is my God, and I trust him."*
> *Psalm 91:2 (NLT)*

Surrendering our fears to God, so that He may do a sanctifying work in us through any experience in life is a reflection of our trust that He truly has our best interest at heart.

In trust, faith, and surrender we need to give Him all of ourselves; all our hopes, dreams, fears, burdens, pains, everything. Like any relationship, our trust in God is developed and revealed over time as we chose to be vulnerable through the tears and the laughter each experience may bring. When one finds loyalty, support, encour-

> *"All you who fear the LORD, trust the LORD! He is your helper and your shield."*
> *Psalm 115:11 (NLT)*

agement, strength, safety, and love from the other in hard times, trust is established and built up. The experience we may encounter on this journey of motherhood is an opportunity for us to grow more intimately in our relationship with Christ, as we trust Him more and more.

We need to view our God as the most wise, most powerful one, worthy of our trust. He is far more powerful than any man. "It is better to take refuge in the LORD than to trust in man," (Psalm 118:8, NLT) Where is our trust in regard to childbirth? Do we trust in ourselves to make all the wise decisions without the counsel or wisdom of the Lord? Or do we trust Him above all men, above all doctors and even midwives? I am not saying not to have their help at all . . . I am asking, in whom do you put your trust? It is fully possible to have a baby

> *"Those who know your name will trust in you, for you, LORD, have never forsaken those who seek you."*
> *Psalm 9:10 (NIV)*

in the hospital and fully and completely trust in and rely on the Lord. Just as it is fully possible for a woman to have a home birth and full rely on and trust in the Lord. The point is to seek to completely trust the Lord. To seek Him in all things to lead us in all our decisions in regards to childbirth. If He leads you toward having a home birth, great. If He leads you to have a hospital birth, great. But is the Lord your trust? Is He the focus? Are you inviting Him to be present and redeem your birth?

Understanding our need for His strength in this process comes from seeking humility. We need to have a clear and biblical perspective on birth, on pain in birth, and then humbly come to the Lord for strength. We can seek humility and ask the Lord to make us women who are humble, loving, and self-controlled. As we seek Him and ask for these righteous attributes, He will give us what we ask. He will provide all we need to bring forth life, gently and gracefully. We can give birth in a way that glorifies our Lord and Savior if we seek to put our trust in Him, humbling recognizing our need for His strength in the birthing process. Then choose to allow the Lord to do a marvelous work in our life, surrendering to the sanctification (growth) God has purposed for us to experience in His grace.

We need to understand that birth is really just another sanctifying event in our life, an opportunity for spiritual growth. After recognizing this opportunity, we need to purposefully choose to work with the Lord, allowing Him to do a work in us. It takes choosing to surrender so that you can grow.

There is no real simple way to express the intimate closeness one can experience with God in the moments of childbirth as you focus on Him and things above, and not on the earthly pain (Col. 3:1). For women who have experienced God and don't have a strong recollection of the pain, this phenomenon is best described by the fact that we as humans cannot truly focus on Jesus and heavenly things while focusing on earthly things simultaneously. While a woman may be consciously aware of the physical pain of birth, when she focuses on God, His promises and blessings, when she is focused on worshipping and in communion with God in prayer, she doesn't focus on the pain. Her mental focus has been shifted toward God. Her paradigm transcends above the physical pain and is fully focused on the Lord. The blessing that comes to the woman who focuses on the Lord in birth is that her perspective on her experience is transformed. While laboring, she isn't focused on the pain, desiring it to be gone and avoided, but rather she is in awe of how good God is and focused on the things above. She is focused on the blessing to come, in the birth of her child. She is focused on how amazing God is to have created her body to do this amazing work. She is experiencing the presence of the Lord in a way like no other, and her faith in Him is strengthened. Once the work is accomplished the sense of satisfaction that comes to the woman who has fully trusted the Lord in this work and experienced Him in all the little and large ways throughout the birth is paramount in her relationship with her Deliverer. This experience has become a milestone to praise the Lord, to remember as an experience of growth, not a horror story. Not an experience one wants to forget.

> "Behold, God is my salvation; I will trust, and will not be afraid; for the LORD GOD is my strength and my song, and he has become my salvation." Isaiah 12:2

This kind of focus doesn't just happen in birth. One cannot just write it down on a birth plan list and assume she won't focus on the pain. Your mind needs mental training to focus on the Lord. Meditating on His Word, in worship, or in prayer are all good ways to train your mind to focus on heavenly things, not earthly circumstances. This is a spiritual discipline that is not just useful in birth but one we should pursue to exhibit in life in general. Your efforts will not be in vain. As a Christian in a fallen world, it is vital we choose to focus on God and not earthly things. If one really approaches pregnancy as a training ground for birth, parenthood, and life in general, it will be a sanctifying experience. A lot of growth will occur.

> "You keep him in perfect peace whose mind is stayed on you, because he trusts in you. Trust in the LORD forever, for the LORD GOD is an everlasting rock." Isaiah 26:3,4

If we as a Christian community pursued getting prepared for this event spiritually and dedicating this time to the Lord, for Him to teach us His ways, imagine how much more prepared parents would be. One can read all the great books available on parenting and childbirth, but if we don't have a relationship with our Lord where He is speaking his truth to us and we believeHis word to be true and then acting in faith and obedience, what good is our faith? God blessed us with much knowledge and truth in regard to childbirth, dealing with trials, suffering, and pain. We only need to live our lives in belief of the truth He has provided.

Preparing your heart for the sanctifying work God may want to do in your life may also require allowing Him to redeem some relationships in your life, and sometimes even in your past. The Lord wants healing in the lives of those who love Him. A key exercise is asking God to reveal to you what relationships He may want to heal through your childbirth (marriage, mother, etc.)?

Ultimately the only way to prepare for the sanctification process one can experience in birth is to simply draw near to the Lord. Start purposefully practicing spiritual disciplines. Pursue God in studying the word, prayer, worship, and service. Seek God alone, not allowing any other human to be an idol in your life.

Deliverance from Pain

The Lord wants to be the one to deliver you from your pain. He wants you to cry out to Him, call on Him, and rely solely on Him and His miraculous strength. I find it so amazing that our bodies we created in such a way that any fear we are struggling with in birth has direct impact on the progress of our labor. That being said, one way our gracious Lord delivers us from more prolonged pain, is through dealing with our fears and allowing God to do a healing work in our lives before birth. If we pursue Him in regard to have a biblical perspective on fear, God in turn fully blesses our life, even in a physical way during our birth experience. When we are truly seeking the Lord in our personal walk with him, He blesses our lives.

The Lord so deeply desires for you to know Him more intimately. And He deeply desires for you to understand more fully His saving power. When a woman fully surrenders all in childbirth, she can and will experience Him as her Deliverer. Lord Jesus, we pray in your name that we might have the strength to be broken and powerless before your throne in the moments of labor and childbirth. Teach us all more about who you are, what you have done for us and what you can do! We surrender our wills, our hopes, and our convictions to you and ask you to refine us and redeem our birth experiences. May we be bonded as sisters in Christ who have experienced You in a deep and profound way in childbirth. Bless all of us Lord, that we may tell the stories of Your deliverance. Amen

> "My comfort in my suffering is this: Your promise preserves my life." Psalm 119:50

What about an Emergency?

No matter where birth takes place, complications may arise that require medical intervention, and I am 100% in support of it in these cases.

As Christians we need to be wise as serpents, and gentle as doves. In regard to our views on childbirth, we also need to use wisdom, not harboring pride. We need to use discretion, not fear. Being in pain is not an emergency. Although sometimes certain types of pain can be a signal that something is wrong, that there is real need for concern. It is important we choose labor partners who have had experience birthing babies. If an emergency arises, they can recognize it and know how to deal with it appropriately. And in those cases, we need to use wisdom and not foolishly reject medical care. In emergencies we need to exercise humility and be willing to surrender the situation unto the Lord. We are so blessed today, that God has allowed the medical field to make the advancements it has made. As I mentioned earlier, mortality rates are directly impacted due to surgeons, hospitals, medical procedures, and advances. In cases of an emergency, we need to receive the help that

> **We need to have a balanced view, recognizing birth is not an emergency, but sometimes emergencies DO happen in birth.**

is available with a thankful heart and submit to their requirements in those situations.

This may mean surrendering a dream or vision of what we hoped for in our births and a willingness to accept whatever lessons God could teach us through this unfortunate event.

When the mother or baby's life is at risk, we are fortunate to have access to surgical techniques that can save lives or prevent serious complications. We need to thankfully accept their help with grace; being aware and observant of the spiritual needs of those around us. Hospitals are full of pain, suffering, and loss, but they are also a place of healing, hope, and miracles. As Christians, we need to try to keep our focus on the Lord; even in those emergencies. It is the hope of the Lord and the promise that He will provide what we need to get through whatever trials we face, that we can trust in Him always. I can't imagine how hard it would be to walk through this life without the Lord, walking through the trials that can occur, without the counsel of His Spirit, the comfort from His hand, the wisdom of His Word, and the love of His Son. Even with the Lord by your side, emergencies are never easy. We are human, and we have times when we even wrestle with God and cry out why? Even in those times, your faith is a witness. When others see your wrestling with a God, they see your faith in a God, when many today don't even have that. Authenticity and sharing where you are and what you are learning is sometimes what another needs to hear to begin a journey of faith in God. And other times simply being in the hospital in a time of trial and responding in the strength of faith can be a witness to others. As we keep our focus on the mission of the cross and His promises, walking through these emergencies becomes more than just about us and more about the big picture, the advancement of the Kingdom.

You're probably thinking, *sounds easy, but so hard to do.* While this book is not about preparing your heart, soul, and mind to deal with an emergency, that is really what it comes down to. How we handle anything in life is truly a reflection of the true condition of all three (heart, soul, and mind). If we are seeking His wisdom in the Word of God and seeking to understand and know more about God, who He is and What He has done, our minds will be more prepared. When we seek God in prayer and we have truly personal and honest relationships with God, our hearts with be more prepared. And when we practice praising Him, worshiping Him, serving Him and seek to really know Him our souls will be more prepared to respond to trials with grace, faith, gratitude, and hope. The more we trust God, out of a reflection of knowing Him, the more easily we will surrender the situation into His hands and allow Him to carry our burdens.

My dear friend Brenda is wonderful examples of shining God's light before men in a hospital through the way she and her husband Karry dealt with an emergency in their life. Brenda and Karry had been married for almost two years and wanted to start a family, but Brenda had two miscarriages. Brenda's heart yearned for a baby, and so they began contemplating adoption. As they began looking into adopting, they found a little boy in Kazakhstan. As the excitement grew toward adopting and their hearts became attached to the idea, the Lord blessed Brenda's womb with their firstborn son, Isaac. I remember how joyful Brenda was to be pregnant, but also nervous she would lose her baby, after having had two miscarriages already. At six months gestation, Brenda began having pre-term labor symptoms, so they sought medical help after trying everything they could. Brenda had to have an emergency cesarean.

"When I learned that my baby was going to be born at twenty-six weeks gestation, I was scared for his life. I did not know if he would live, or if he survived, what kind of quality of life he might have. It was an incredibly scary day. I had an emergency C-section, and my sweet baby did not cry, and I did not get to really see him for about four or five hours.

At that time, were new to our church and a young families' group through our church and everyone rallied around us and encouraged us and prayed for us and for our tiny baby boy. Their prayers and physical support (like visiting us, helping us clean our home, and making us meals while we spent so many days at the hospital) were what kept us going.

I remember being just so happy that our son was alive. I knew there would be challenges ahead of him, and that his life was fragile, but I remember feeling an amazing sense of peace. I just knew God was going to take care of him and protect his tiny (1 lb. 12 oz.) life. One of the nurses said to me, condescendingly, 'Oh, you're the optimistic one I heard about.' I can only hope that the optimism (or; faith in God's plans for our son!) was a testimony to the great God we worship!

It was weird to be in a place where I had zero power to fix anything. I think God had me there on purpose! I had to learn to trust in Him, because He was ALL I had to trust in. As amazing as my husband is, there was nothing he could do to keep our son alive and well. As educated and experienced as the many nurses and doctors were, they were only human beings with finite knowledge and abilities. There was nobody in our life who could fix this situation. God was IT, and I had to trust in Him! Because of that experience, I think I learned a deeper trust in God than I had ever experienced before.

I wrote out my husband's favorite passage, Psalm 84, and taped it up on our son's incubator, where he lived for the first three months of his life. Psalm 84:5a says, "Blessed are those whose strength is in you," and I am so thankful He brought us to a place where our only strength was in Him! We had no strength to offer up for our son, it was all God's! Psalm 84:12 says, "LORD Almighty, blessed is the one who trusts in you." We certainly learned to trust in Him, and He definitely blessed us for trusting Him!

While we were in the hospital we met another family who were not Christians. They too had a daughter in the NICU. We developed a life-long relationship with them from our time together there. To this day we still get together with them every couple of months and my son Isaac prays for their daughter and other children every night. I even remember watching Isaac showing their daughter the Bible during one of our play dates (they were only two years old). God is so good that He even uses my little boy, whom we could have lost, to witness to other little children. God is worthy to be praised."

Before all of these unfortunate events occurred Brenda and I had been hosting a neighborhood play date luncheon in our homes as an outreach in attempts to create community (since we lived just a few blocks from each other). Not many were believers and I remember how much of an impact Brenda's faith and joy had on those women. Many of the women were Muslim, and they were amazed at her joy as they watched from with a bird's eye view what they walked through.

When Isaac was five months old and having only been home from the hospital for two months, Brenda became pregnant again. Since she had such an early delivery with Isaac, the doctors performed a cervical cerclage and put Brenda on full bed rest at four months along. What a blessing to have another baby on the way, but what a physically and emotionally difficult season, to have a high needs infant at the same time as being on bed-rest. Karry, her husband, is and was an amazing support to her, juggling work with serving (through cooking, taking them to doctor's appointments, etc.) her and their son every minute he wasn't at work. The church and Brenda's family were also supportive as they spent many hours helping take care of them (both Isaac and Brenda) so Karry could work. Kaleb, their second son, was born early, but he was healthy. After having these two emergencies, doctors recommended not having more children biologically, but God had placed a desire on Brenda and Karry's hearts for a large family. They have adopted two more children, are foster care parents, and are planning to adopt more children. God has truly created in them a capacity to handle a lot more than most people could ever imagine. They have grown spiritually to a place of being able to do this because God has prepared them through these trials.

You see their unfortunate events had eternal purposes:

- Their hearts grew open to the idea of adoption and now they have two adopted and are pursuing adopting more.
- God used them to witness to the nurses and doctors as well as other families while they were in the hospital.

- They developed a lifelong friendship with a non-believing family and continue to love them with God's love.
- Their situation provided an avenue for the church to serve them and be blessed by doing so.
- The women in our neighborhood were impacted by Brenda's faith and confidence in God that everything would be ok. They were blessed to be able to serve her with meals when she was on bed rest.
- Brenda and Karry's faith and trust in God were tested, and they were blessed spiritually for having faith in Him.

There are many different kinds of lessons that can be learned, and opportunities we miss when we don't purpose to keep our eyes on Jesus as we walk through trials in life. Everyone's testimony is a bit different, but just as Job was tested and lost everything, he wrestled with the truth, and he still praised God and didn't lose faith. In the end, God blessed Job and honored him by telling his story in the Bible. We have been given an example of how to deal with trials in life; we need to approach them with the same intentionality and trusting abandon.

For those in the church who hold to a more extreme view that home birth is the only way to have babies, I would like to speak a word of truth to you. Home births can be an immense blessing within the life of a woman and the life of a family, but God is everywhere. By believing only God can be at a home birth, one is putting God in a box. He is everywhere, at all times, and can be experienced by anyone at any place. Sometimes life is hard; sometimes there are emergencies, even in birth. When an individual has given her life to God, she can trust He is in control. Since He is omniscient and omnipotent, we can have confidence He has allowed this circumstance. Since the circumstance or emergency is inevitable, we need to embrace our faith in these times of need. Allow Him to be in charge, not our standards or expectations. We need to lean on Christ, allow Him to be our strength as we deal with whatever outcome we experience. We need to be willing to let Him mold us and teach us.

When I was first writing this chapter, I thought to myself, "If I were to ever experience an emergency in birth, I would hope in that moment I would be looking for God to make clear His path, however hard that may be. Whether that be witnessing to a nurse or doctor, living my faith out trusting Him, or allowing my faith in Him to grow and my children to learn as they watch." Then I looked back for a moment and realized I have had three pregnancies when doctors suggested we terminate pregnancy, one child who was born with trachea malasia (who stopped breathing at twenty-four hours old), one baby born with a hole in his heart, and a benign mixed tumor removed from the side of my face. When you see God's sovereignty and experience Him by your side through it all, when all is said and done, you don't view life's experiences as an emergency. Trials may come in this life, for some of us it may be in birth, for many, most likely (statistically) it will not. In those trials we are faced with an option. We have a option to carry that burden ourselves, to close off, get angry with God or others (hospital staff), or we can realize life brings its trials and that this is out of our control, prayerfully submit it unto God the Father, and allow the learning to begin gracefully.

Let's be Thankful

Years ago when a woman was experiencing an emergency, often the outcome was death, either of the mother or the baby. And if not death, pain, physical limitations, and disabilities were common. Today we are so blessed that in these cases, we can accept the help of professionals who are trained in how to treat emergencies. There is still much we don't understand about birth, and even more we don't have direct control over. In some cases, despite a woman's best efforts to have a natural, undisturbed birth, complications arise that require medical attention (and transfer to a hospital if she started laboring at home). In these circumstances, I absolutely endorse taking advantage of whatever interventions may protect the health and safety of both the mother and baby. At the end of the day, that is far, far more important than the method by which the baby was born.

We need to have a healthy view of childbirth and emergencies. Clearly, with technology what it is today and the knowledge that both midwives and ob-gyns bring to the childbirth arena, most high-risk pregnancies can be evaluated in early pregnancy. I am not a professional who evaluates emergencies and would never claim to be. The reality we live with today is that emergencies do happen, and they are usually not something one can expect, hence the name emergency. Some do know ahead of time, others won't know until they are in the midst of it. Regardless of the type of emergency, as Christian women, we need to have faith and trust in God, asking Him for a new kind of strength, a strength to trust Him, a strength to surrender maybe even the dream we had of our births, allowing God to do a different sanctifying work in us. All things, even bad situations can reflect the goodness of our father if we look for them. We just need to train ourselves to look for the good.

When I had my post-partum hemorrhage after giving birth to Ethan, I lost over half of my blood. I went from a 14.4 hemoglobin level to a 7.1 a week AFTER birth. There were moments when I was in and out of consciousness as I was trying my best to make it through four hours of intense contractions when I birthed three huge clots almost the size of my baby. It was intense and scary, especially for my husband. Looking back though, I am thankful for so many things. I am thankful for my midwives and how they treated me. They knew all the homeopathic and natural methods to help me get through it, they were right there with me the whole way. I know without a doubt in my mind I was exactly where God wanted me for that birth and that those midwives were trained and knew exactly how to help me.

After my hemorrhage and arrival back home, I was on bed rest for about four weeks to rebuild my red blood cells. It wasn't easy. In fact I struggled a lot, both emotionally and physically. I couldn't stand for more than two minutes without getting dizzy and my feet swelling up like balloons. Emotionally, I was concerned about my other children, and what a sacrifice this was for our whole family to have to take care of me. I thought that was my job, and I so badly wanted to do my job well. Looking back though, I know God allowed me to go through what I went through, not just for my refining but also for my family's refining. Sometimes the emergencies or accidents or health issues that happen to us end up being a growth time for someone else close to us as well. In this case, the blessing was abundant. All of my children had the opportunity to care for me, their new baby brother, dad, and each other in ways they hadn't before. I was forced to have to sit back and let them do it all.

During this time I was humbled as my nine-year-old daughter was treating me by feeding me chlorophyll/coconut milk mixture and juicing kale and amaranth. She got to laugh as I forced down the floradix (iron & herb supplement). She was learning, more than I even knew. She loved it and grew so much. All of my children helped with all kinds of things around the house and with their younger siblings. There was a spirit of unity and teamwork becoming our way of life in such a grander scale. Our church was such a blessing to us as they prayed for our family, brought meals, and took care of us as much as they could. My mother also came and lived with us for a week so my husband could go on a business trip. She served my kids, played with them, and she lifted my spirits as she encouraged me when I was feeling low. All in all, the growth wasn't all for me. Every one of us grew because I couldn't just do it myself, like I always had. It was humbling, but so good. I wouldn't take back those four weeks of cuddling with my sixth child in bed constantly for anything. It allowed me to bond with my new baby in ways I might not have had if I were up and at 'em right away.

We need to look hard for the hidden blessings that can come out of a journey of suffering and trials. When we are able to see those blessings, then we can praise Him and give Him the glory. Then the enemy has no power over the circumstance that happened in our lives. That should be our fight, to find the good even when it may not seem like there is any. Choosing to be thankful and focus on the blessing, acknowledging how great it was that the medical field was able to help, and that in the end we have a healthy baby and mom.

If our hearts are transformed to be more like our Father in Heaven, we will begin to see every child as a gift and blessing from Him, regardless of how or where the baby was born. My hope is that any one reading this would seek God in regard to inviting His presence into their birth experiences, regardless of where they have their babies and regardless of their circumstances.

If the Lord allows us to walk through emergency experiences in our births, we need to look to Him, we need to lean on Him, and look for the ways in which we can glorify Him where He has placed us at that moment. What lessons in life can we learn from our experience and how can we build up others through our testimony?

> "Though the fig tree should not blossom, nor fruit be on the vines the produce of the olive fail and the fields yield no food, the flock be cut off from the fold and there be no herd in the stalls, yet I will rejoice in the Lord; I will take joy in the God of my salvation. God, the Lord, is my strength; he makes my feet like the deer's; he makes me tread on my high places. To the choirmaster: with stringed instruments." Hab. 3:17-19

Throughout Scripture we have been given examples of ordinary men and women who have chosen in the moments of trial to rejoice in the Lord and to look for the good and praise Him even when there is no good to be found by man's eyes. They are our examples. This is what we, as women, should strive to do if we are faced with an emergencies. God is still there with you, ready to provide all you need.

Praising God in the emergency can be difficult, even more difficult can be choosing to search for the refining lesson that can be found and experienced in the process. Sometimes, the Lord allows us to go through these experiences in life for more than ourselves. When I was on bed rest with my last two births and in pain, it was very difficult for all of those around me, who love me, to watch me go through what I did physically. For some of them it was very challenging for their faith. By the end of this season though, there was growth, spiritual growth and relational growth.

For some, the lesson and refinement to be experienced is so intimate and personal because it takes great pains to learn the lesson or to actually surrender. Women who experience emergency birth operations can struggle to find the good in what they experienced. They often experience massive trauma because the process of dealing with the reality of their situations is so humbling and hard to walk through. Of course, there are all kinds of emotions playing into it as well. If there is a case where a baby is in danger, the mother can feel out of control, not being able to care for her baby immediately as her instincts are telling her to. This can be very traumatic.

Then there are times when the emergency itself can do a spiritually refining process in a woman's spiritual life, a refining process where even idols may be in need of being crucified.

Crucifying Idols

"My dream was to be forty-five years old, but look twenty-five. I wanted to show my six boys you could be healthy and pregnant, even in your forties. I dreamt of showing my teenage sons what it meant to be this Proverbs 31 woman who could do it all. Cheer on soccer games, do worship team, home school, and have another baby, even at forty-five. I had one future daughter- in-law at the time, and I had so anticipated including her in this intimate experience, so as to teach her and model for her how special home birth could be. I wanted to show my boys that if you eat well, get physical exercise, and do everything you should naturally, you could have a healthy birth and healthy baby, and everything will turn out just as planned. Looking back, I think I even wanted to make a statement to my children that having a large family was doable. I wanted our sons to see their dad and me enjoying and welcoming this late-in-life baby to our family. After having six natural births at home, I had no intention of having a hospital birth at all."

Doesn't it all sound perfect, the vision of a strong woman, fully confident in her ability to give birth and in God's design? She wanted to purposefully model motherhood to her sons and future daughter-in-law. But God had another plan for Julie and her family. God wanted to sanctify Julie more. Though giving birth naturally can be a very sanctifying experience, for Julie, God knew what was best. His best was not a home birth. Julie was forced to submit all her hopes and dreams to God.

"I was not at all in a place of willingly submitting to the reality of the situation. From a psychological perspective, I was in denial."

Julie's blood pressure was out the roof. After her thirty-six week check up, her midwife told Julie she wouldn't feel comfortable performing a home birth and that she needed to see a doctor and go to the hospital. Determined to have a natural home birth, Julie and her husband sought out a local naturopathic doctor who performed home births. He also turned Julie away. "If you or I had blood pressure that high right now, we would both be dead," the doctor told Peter. At that moment, there was no doubt in Peter's mind, he knew he would need to gently lead his wife to the hospital. Panicked, Julie tried to make excuses to go home . . . '"I need my toothbrush, clothes, things for the baby." In a loving and gentle tone, Peter said, "No Julie, we need to go to the hospital now."

"In hindsight, every expectation I had for Simon's birth went out the window. All those dreams of modeling a healthy birth to my sons were gone. When in reality what was modeled for them was what did happen, as husband and wife. What we did show them was the reality of what it looks like for a man to take care of his wife. I admit I fought it tooth and nail. I did not want to go to that hospital. As we sat in the parked car for a few moments before going in, I just wept. Then Peter got out and opened the door for me. I got out and stood in front of the door to the hospital. I began thinking of all the things I was about to lose, and I would turn around and head back to the car. Peter again would gently coax me toward the hospital doors, then again I would be reminded of all my expectations, my ideal birth situation, and again I would turn around and head back to the car.

After time and time again of heading back and forth to the doors of the hospital, thinking of all my intentions for strengthened relationships, and the intimacy with my Lord, finally I had to submit. I submitted myself physically, but my mind and heart were hard and unwavering. I was angry, mad, and upset with Peter. I didn't know why he was doing this to me.

While waiting in the hospital before the procedure, we talked, we prayed, we cried. Coming to the decision to have a C-section wasn't an easy one. I couldn't actually say the words, 'Let's have a caesarean,' so he made the decision. Our sons came in and dear friends the Harris family came in and waited with us. We sang hymns, talked and prayed, which brought me some peace. Sono, a dear sister in the Lord, grabbed my arm and reassured me, 'God is sovereign even when things don't go as we planned. He is using them for your good and His glory.' She confronted me with another truth there in that hospital as well, when she gently said, 'This is going to give you so much more compassion for other women.' She was right; this was probably one of the purposes God had for me to learn through this experience.

As I was getting prepared to go into the surgery room my worst nightmare began to happen. I felt like I was being crucified. They actually tied down my arms with straps just as Jesus' arms were tied down. The thought of the doctor cutting my abdomen open was freaking me out. I wanted to kick and scream, but I knew I had to surrender. I had to submit to my husband's wishes and the doctor's recommendation.

I wasn't happy. I am always happy at my births, but this time I was overcome with anger. My body submitted, but my heart did not. The emotional disappointment was too much for me to bear. I hadn't even made optional birth plans. They weren't even something I thought about; that's how strong willed I was.

After the procedure was over, I was still mad and had a hard time adjusting. There was frustration with not being able to nurse right away because he had to be in the nursery. Losing that closeness I was so used to and anticipating was killing my spirit. The hospital could not be compared to having a baby at home. It took me months to come to grips with what had happened. I kept thinking on how all my dreams and expectations were crucified. Even then I don't think I fully got over it.

Submission to my husband, well, let's just say this was one of the toughest times for me to fully submit to my husband. I really didn't want to. Looking back, looking for a reason to justify this experience, I wonder, 'Was this preparation for letting sons go to public high school?' I remember after the birth, asking my husband, 'Why did you do this to me?' He kindly replied, 'I wanted you to be around to raise this son with me.' I thought he was against me, but in that moment I realized he was thinking of my best interests. He was loving and protecting me. That was what was being modeled for my six sons. I realize now that this was so much bigger than being just about me; there was something in this experience for everyone."

Things don't always go the way we plan them to go. We need to be open to God's wisdom, trusting Him in ways we haven't trusted Him before. In reality, there was a crucifixion happening: Julie's idols. There is a real temptation for us to make idols out of things such as natural childbirth or home birth. Just as there is a temptation for us to make an idol out of how many children we have or what kind of career we have. God does not want us to have any idols. He is a jealous God, who wants all of our heart. He doesn't want our hearts to grow hardened toward others because of an idol like natural childbirth. He alone deserves our worship and respect. He alone deserves our loyalty and trust.

That day as Julie was lying on the operating table with her arms stretched out and tied down, her idols were crucified. She could no longer hold them so precious and dear. He was refining her to be more like Him, merciful, compassionate, loving, and faithful.

"Honestly, I look at my past experience with Simon's birth and I think I am still learning all God had for me to learn through why he allowed it to happen that way. But I know God is good and I trust Him."

What lesson can we learn from Julie's testimony? We need to learn from the Titus 2 women in our lives. As they tell their stories and about what the Lord has taught them, we need to learn from their examples, lest we go through a similar experience in life. The warning I glean from Julie is this: we need to be careful not to put natural childbirth or home birth on a pedestal. This is a perfect example of how God did a sanctifying work in Julie, her marriage, and her family through Simon's birth, even though it was by c- section. It isn't the act of pushing out a baby that is sanctifying. It is the experience of having to surrender and submit to God, whatever His will is for your birth, whether that be a thirty-eight hour labor, or a four hour labor, or a C-section. Ultimately we are to seek Him in all things.

We also need to be careful as we are preparing to birth our babies, not to be walking pride fully as though we have it all together. Instead, we should be focusing our time on preparing our hearts for whatever the Lord may have in store for us, so that when the test or trial comes our way, because it will eventually. We will be ready. Ready to submit. Ready to let the Lord lead.

I also loved how she shared honestly about her struggle in submitting to her husband because I think many of us can relate. Even though her heart wasn't there, she physically submitted out of the knowledge God wanted her to submit. It took her time, but her heart finally followed and she understood her husband was just protecting her.

In the chapter titled "Birth Can Bless Your Marriage," we engage how important it is to allow your husband to be the protector in your relationship. How submission is God's design for your protection. I believe this concept is critical in the case of an emergency. Sometimes the husband has a clearer vision of the truth within a given situation, especially if the woman has envisioned and dreamt of her perfect birth or is even simply in denial. In these circumstances, I believe submission or obedience and surrender to the truth that is being spoken is critical. God has chosen for you and your husband to be a team, even in birth. As women seeking to glorify God and follow His Word, we need to follow the heads of our households. We need to allow our husbands to speak into our lives in regard to these kinds of decisions. God knew who would be the best protector and provider for YOU! Allow your husband to do his job. He will be held accountable before God one day for how he did in that arena. Choose to make his job a little easier. If your husband does not have peace about having a home birth, pray about it together, but ultimately, do not let it become an area of division.

Allow this experience to be one where your marriage can be strengthened in that you put faith and trust in your husband's decision to love and protect you. And be thankful you have a husband who is dealing in reality and loves you so deeply, as though loving himself, that he wants what is best for you and your baby. Be thankful simply, for him.

> *"Wives submit to your husbands, as is fitting to the Lord. Husbands, love your wives and do not be harsh with them."*
> **Col 3:18-19**

Can God be in your experience if you have an epidural?

Yes, He can. Just because you choose to have pain medication doesn't mean God checks out. God is always with us, waiting for the invitation to be active in our lives. For those who have epidurals, while you may not experience exactly the same as what those women who choose to have natural birth do, you can still plan and purpose to have worship music and prayer as your focus. You can still choose to involve your children as much as you wish. You can still experience growth in your marriage. The birth of a baby, no matter how it takes place, is a spiritual experience because God created this miracle, this blessing. What a joyous time for any couple to have their family growing. Remember, God is bigger than epidurals and if your heart's desire is truly to experience Him, you will.

> *"In this same way husbands ought to love their wives as their own bodies. He who loves his wife loves himself."*
> **Eph. 5:28**

> *"Husbands, in the same way be considerate as you live with your wives, and treat them with respect as the weaker partner and as heirs with you of the gracious gift of life, so that nothing will hinder your prayers."* **1 Peter 3:7**

My prayer is that you would be encouraged more than anything by a new confidence in how God designed your body to do this marvelous work. In being encouraged, I pray you would purposefully engage inviting Jesus and the presence of the Holy Spirit to be there with you. That your relationship with Him would be strengthened and equip you for all that life has in store for you.

Don't Judge

Within the church there is the temptation to judge one another on both sides of the gap (see chapter one). Women who have had epidurals feel judged by those who have had natural births. Those who have had natural births feel judged by those who have had epidurals. Then there are the women who have had emergency caesareans and even those who have had caesareans for the sake of wanting to avoid any kind of pain, schedule their babies' birthdays, and have it all done in a half hour. Ladies, may I just call out this battle? Judging never profited anyone. What we need is for there to be biblical teaching by Titus 2 women on the topic of childbirth, from a heart of love, to want to equip and teach, help walk beside, give confidence when it is needed, but NOT to judge. Women coming along side women, mothers coming along side daughters, and speaking truth in love. We need a paradigm shift towards trusting God more in ALL things, including birth. There needs to be women doing this, then standing up praising God and leading and loving.

I have personally experienced women labeling me as one of "them" just because they know I have had six children, all natural births, and I home educate. Somehow they justify that they know what I believe without ever asking, just because of stereotyping and judging. Maybe they have met judgmental women before. Whatever the case, they themselves are judging and comparing. We need to be careful not to bring division among believers because of how we have done it. We need not judge our sisters to justify our own actions, either way. For women who experience feeling judged because of having an epidural or cesarean, my heart goes out to you. I grieve that you have felt judged. I have felt that same feeling for having babies naturally. May I speak a word of encouragement to you: do not stop doing what the Lord has called you to do based on feeling judged. The best decision for your family is the one that helps you to trust in God and glorify Him best, whatever that may be.

In many church environments, the topic of encouraging young women, teaching them and living by example, sharing their personal faith journeys through what they have learned in birth, has been very minimal, if at all. I urge you older women to be open and vulnerable for the Lord to use you and your testimonies to encourage the younger women to seek God in their experience and to surrender to learning whatever He wants to teach them personally.

Why are we so afraid to teach on this? I believe we are afraid of being called judgmental, but God wants us to simply encourage one another in all things, including childbirth. We need to love everyone, and not judge what they do, or how they give birth, but to pray for one another for the health of the mother and baby, but also for God to make Himself known, that He may be glorified in their births. This is a milestone in every woman's life. Let's help prepare our younger sisters for this amazing experience so they may get more out of it!

As a church body we need to be focused on uplifting women in their faith journeys and equipping mothers to seek God, have faith, and to listen to His guidance in making ANY decision. Then after doing so, we need to fully support whatever decision they make, as Jesus calls us to.

It Doesn't Matter Where You Have Your Baby!

Inviting the Lord and experiencing His presence can happen anywhere: home, hospital, or birth center. God doesn't live in a box. We cannot put a lid on His power and presence. It is a foundational doctrinal belief that He is omnipresent, everywhere at all times.

I had my first four babies in a hospital, and I can share with you, that even though I personally prefer birth center, for me, my hospital births were just as spiritual. They were just different, but then every birth is completely unique in its own right anyway. I will say though, I had to purpose, plan, and be more determined to have a relaxed atmosphere. It is simply, much less work to have your baby in a quiet, familiar place.

In our experiences, God always blessed us with at least one Christian birth attendant who encouraged us to stay the course with our heart's desires and advocated for us all our desires for our births. Beyond that though, there was clearly a reason why we had our babies where and how we had them. God made Himself known to us clearly each time and I am ever so grateful.

We should not have a view that hospitals, doctors, midwives, or doulas are evil or the wrong caregivers or incapable caregivers. It is truly an individual issue with many variables. We should be thankful for all of these caregivers and the different gifts they bless us with.

There are many fantastic women who serve daily in hospitals who are Christians and those women are so blessed when strong Christian women come in and glorify God in their labors and births. It not only encourages their faith but also helps them be a witness with other nurses, doctors, and midwives on staff when they can share live stories of faith. As the body of Christ, we need to recognize that because life and death are not all about us, neither are all of our experiences. When you are fully surrendered to God and ask Him to expand your territory to serve Him in making disciples of all nations, be aware you may be called to have a hospital birth simply to witness. Who knows? That is something you will need to ask the Lord. Ultimately, you can purpose to create whatever atmosphere in your room you want. If you surrender it to Jesus in prayer and you invite Him, focusing on Him He will be there. He is there.

In regard to division in the church and even our society, there are two perspectives most prevalent today. There is the belief (lie) that you aren't fully trusting God if you don't have a home birth. Others believe home births are foolish and testing God (also a lie). May I just say that judging where others choose to give birth is such a waste of time and energy. It's like judging other peoples' educational choices for THEIR children. It is not our jurisdiction to make decisions for others. We are privileged to have the freedom to make these decisions in the first place, and I believe we are more blessed because of it. Can't our faith be grown by acknowledging the good and God in home births, birth center births, and hospital births? Isn't it strengthening to know God has no boundaries?

This is an area within the Christian community where we have the opportunity to exercise grace.

For some, God may lay a deep passion on the couples' hearts to have a birth at home, where it is quiet and intimate. They may be planning for this event to be a special time at home, either by themselves or with family. Whichever they decide, they have their reasons. For some who may choose to have their babies at the hospital, it may be because they have an insurance company that won't pay for any care unless they do that, so in order to be wise with their money and not to go into debt to have a homebirth, they choose that avenue. Maybe there is a perceived issue with mama or baby and to take precautions they decide to have the baby at the hospital. Or maybe, just maybe, God knows a doctor or a nurse in that hospital who needs to be witnessed to by the example of a strong couple welcoming a gift from the Lord in a way that glorifies Him.

These are just a few of the variables that can impact a couple in regard to choosing where to deliver their baby. We need to have grace, understanding that **God is everywhere all the time, and God is good all the time.**

Is it harder to worship God in a hospital than at home?

It will be different for everyone. You and your husband need to really pray and seek God as to what kind of birth you want, and take into consideration how you like to worship and birth as well as what your family is comfortable with. There is no formula for having a spiritual birth anywhere. God is simply everywhere. It is just a matter of intentionally inviting Him and preparing your soul to experience Him in a new way. By prepare, I mean, in your birth plan you should include things such as your Bible, specific verses or prayers if you want those read to you aloud, any worship music should be ready to go to lead you in worship when you are struggling to focus on yourself, etc. When you are at home, you have to plan those things out as well, but for many, because they are home, it is easier to worship out loud. The neat thing is God made us all so different and because we are different we glorify Him differently too.

I personally have no problem worshiping anywhere or at any time. I love to worship and I really don't care what other people think because my worship is not for them anyway, it is for my God. It is the same with prayer. But there are those people who are much more conscious of others around them. For those people, they might prefer home birth. The point is we were all made different to beautifully shine our lights for Jesus in the way He made us.

It doesn't matter how you have your baby, with epidural or no epidural!

Your salvation or whether you are a Christian or not is not determined by how you have your baby either. I need to make clear that though I do believe the most natural approach to birth is natural birth, I also do firmly believe God can still be fully present and fully bless a marriage and those involved in the birth when utilizing medications. I would never want to put God in a box to stay He couldn't. However, I do believe strongly in His design of our bodies to perform the function of bringing forth life, and I do believe the facts that when women have epidurals they themselves are limited in their physical abilities to feel and work through the birth process fully aware of what is happening to them. Medicine is typically used for illness and emergency. My personal view of birth is that it is not an illness or an emergency. We were made by God with this ability, although sometimes emergencies do happen in birth.

Nonetheless, having an epidural does not make a woman less of a Christian or less of a mother. We need to guard our hearts against this judgmental lie. We need to recognize nothing we do can ever make us more of a Christian. Our human nature wants to puff itself up. It is the first sin of all mankind to want to be equal to God in knowledge and power. We need to recognize our sinful desire to be powerful or praised and flee from it. We need to be careful not to allow lies to make us self-righteous. Instead we need to encourage one another with truth, pursue godliness, and holiness together, encouraging one another to pursue Him in all things and pursue allowing Him to sanctify us.

I believe within the body of Christ there is a need for some women to be sanctified and grow in understanding that it is okay for women not to have natural birth. It is not an eternal issue. It is not a matter of salvation, nor should it be an issue of division among the women in the church.

We are so quick to make idols out of lesser gods. In the wilderness it was a golden calf, for some women today it is natural birth or home birth. We need to be aware and cautious not to allow any god to distract us from the one true God. We need to be careful not to allow idols in our lives create division among sisters. We need not worship natural birth or home birth. We need to worship the one WHO creates and births the babies: God.

The Main Point

Regardless of how you birth your baby, the point of *Redeeming Childbirth* is to take your journey toward motherhood to the Lord beforehand. Prepare your heart, soul, mind, marriage, family, and relationship with Christ for this experience. Grow in your relationship with Him, and seek His mission for your life and this short but powerful journey you are on. Allow the holy Scriptures to encourage you and equip you for birth and motherhood. Pray and ask God to reveal His mission for you. Discuss it with your husband, and together seek God. Then obey what you feel He is calling you to.

As Christians, regardless of what other women believe about birth or what their experiences were, this is between you and God. If you approach it the way you feel God is revealing to you, then obey Him. Not for anyone else, not for brownie points with God, because He doesn't work on a points system. Seek Him and He will provide all you need spiritually, whether that means having a natural birth, a hospital birth, or experiencing an emergency. God can and will be with you, just ask Him to be. Invite Jesus.

Do not let the where or the how distract you from experiencing His presence and hearing Him reveal His plan for you and your family because it will look different and beautiful from those around you. Focus on Him and truly grasp the concept of being on a mission to learn the lessons He has for you through this experience.

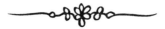

Let's pray

Lord, I pray You would make Your will known to my sister here. Let us all examine our own hearts for any idols we may have and help us not to grow prideful after having experienced You in such an amazing way. I pray You would teach us to trust You and believe you are everywhere with us all the time. I pray our children would see us believing that truth and desire to believe it as well. Lord, help us to be wise in our decision making, not foolish. Help us to use wisdom for our own personal life situations alone, not getting distracted by what others might think of us. Lord, help us to grow in You and purpose to glorify You and magnify You wherever we give birth. May we be a light that shines your glory and bless those around us with your joy and peace.

Thank You for always being there for us; please help us to focus on You. Amen

The Mission of Birth

Already . . . Megan was just nine and a half months old and I was feeling that normal squeamish feeling that sends me to the pharmacy for a pregnancy test. This was our fourth pregnancy, all of the symptoms of pregnancy kicked right into gear, almost as if they had never gone away. With the births of my last two babies being so fresh in my mind, I couldn't help but begin preparing as soon as I found out. I knew my morning sickness was going to kick in full throttle soon, so I wanted to get as caught up and mentally prepared as possible. Choosing the birthplace was easy; I didn't really have any options. Our health insurance was very limited due to the fact that my husband was self-employed, and because of his policy, I either had to have the baby at the hospital or they wouldn't cover any of it, and that included not paying for an emergency. It was the company's way of controlling the chance of a more expensive situation. I was accustomed to this policy, as this was the case with our first three births as well. Having had three babies at the hospital and still experiencing God in such an intimate way, I was okay with this, especially since our first two babies were born with genetic health issues. It was the reality that I need to submit my dreams to; although, I had always desired to have a home birth.

During my second trimester, my family went through a trauma. My father was deathly ill and the doctors were unable to diagnose him for days. As my family waited and watched my dad slowly begin to die, I was overwhelmed with emotion, and rightfully so. The next five months were intense as he was diagnosed with a rare dental related infection called endocarditis. It had spread creating vegetation on his heart that required open-heart surgery. We went through one roller coaster after another as more health issues arose. All we could do was pray and wait. We lived in the ICU for weeks, then in other jurisdictions of the hospital, sleeping on benches, empty hospital beds, and floors. After his heart surgery, he was released to come home which was a huge blessing, but then just one week later, on the Fourth of July, he suffered a stroke. The endocarditis had gone to his brain and created an aneurism. That night everything changed again. Less than two months before my due date, I found myself sleeping in the hospital again. Our family became closer and tighter than ever before. We circled around in the hospital with about fifteen to twenty friends from our churches in the lobby of the hospital and we prayed. We prayed for a miracle, for God to save my father. The surgeons had given my dad a 10% survival rate and we still clung to that hope as the surgeons did what they did best. We dedicated my dad to the Lord asking Him to revive him and use him for His service. Then after hours of surgery and waiting the neurosurgeon came down to say he had made it and that the brain started to swell just as he was removing the skull. My dad was alive. The surgeon was shocked and had no scientific explanation for this miracle and success. Thus began our ministry in the hospital as a family.

Over the months, I came to the realization that my dad had a long road of recovery ahead of him. He was paralyzed on his left side completely, and we were told he would never walk or play guitar again (which was his passion). We took shifts as family members as much as possible to stay with him. We grew close through this trial and we tried to offer comfort to other families we met in the waiting rooms in the ICU and share the testimony of what God had done in my father's life. We had many opportunities to share about our faith, almost daily as we would read aloud the Bible to dad so he could hear the words of the Lord, praying over him while he was in a comma, praying with him before and after surgeries, we grew very close. A few nurses on staff grew to love my dad, and we grew to love them. Our family grew stronger those few months.

During these months of spending so much time at the hospital, my pregnancy began to fly by. I wasn't able to focus on preparing like I had in the past, but God was doing a different kind of preparing in my heart. I had been learning about shining your light for Jesus in the hospitals among the staff. As we had been practically living there, my mom, my dad and I all had had very significant spiritual conversations with care givers there at the hospital and were able to share the love of Christ with them. This kind of became a second nature to me, as I would head to my hospital for my prenatal appointments. In a weird kind of way, hospitals kind of felt like home to me because I had been spending so much time there. I really began to see every hospital staff person as a unique caring person, who had dedicated his or her life to serving others, and I wanted to show them respect for that. So I began purposefully engaging the nurses and midwives who cared for me.

After all, they all knew me well since I was there so frequently. A few of them called me "Fertile Myrtle" because I had had four kids in six years. A few knew me as the only lady ever to give birth under water in their hospital (I had a tub brought in against policy, hehe). Within the first two visits with the midwife, she began asking me more personal questions about faith and size of family, contraceptives, and so on. This particular midwife had been there for my second son's birth and had witnessed much of what we experienced in that birth. She wasn't a believer, but I had known her for about three and a half years, so I shared with her my beliefs and she simply listened. During that visit, the Lord impressed something extremely deep to His heart on mine.

As I thought through all of my birth experiences up to that point, I realized I had been so focused on myself, embracing the experience and ME experiencing His presence, that I was missing out on something. Something so extremely close to God's heart: world missions. Many people view world missions as overseas missions, but I view missions as anywhere in the world. Today the world is scattered abroad and I believe there are just as many lost souls here in America as almost anywhere. I have personally done overseas missions and am very convinced of our need to go as Christians, but I am equally convinced of our need to be intentional wherever God has put us at any given point. Sadly, the harvest is hard here. It is hard being a missionary in your own town because people truly know all about you and your history. But that is what should shine the most: people seeing the change in you, in your heart.

Be a Missionary Wherever You Are

Hudson Taylor once said, "God uses men who are weak and feeble enough to lean on him." When we are in birth, we can come to a place where we are weak and we need to lean on Him. In doing this, we can show doctors, midwives, and nurses an example of Christ working in us; they have the opportunity to walk through a testimony with us. We can be missionaries right where God has placed us. I believe what we need is the church stepping up, to go overseas and to be missionaries here in the work place, neighborhoods, hospitals, and churches of America. We are

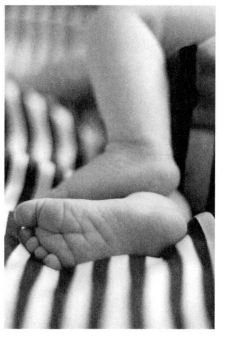

all missionaries; we are all called to the Great Commission. God clearly wants to save even those living here. He is sending missionaries from other countries to America because we have a truly large lost people group.

The reality is most American Christians really truly are guilty of compartmentalizing Jesus. We do it without even thinking about it. If we became more balanced (not compartmentalizing) and integrated our faith into every area of our lives (including birth) and we intentionally began being a missionary wherever God takes us, then we could see a revival in our land.

It is going to take the Body of Christ, stepping out and taking action without timidity and actually living what we believe in every area of our lives to make a difference in this world. The Holy Spirit moves people's hearts, that is not our job, but we do have a responsibility in the advancement of the Kingdom of God. Let's choose to be missionaries in the hospitals, in the birth centers, and in our homes with unbelieving midwives. Let's lay down our pride and pick up the cross of Jesus and get intentional.

As I thought on this, I asked myself, was I purposing to shine my light for Jesus in this place where it is so sterile and in some ways seems spirit-less? Was I on mission? As I sat in my car, listening to worship music, it dawned on me. Just as I had been so passionate about pursuing world missions as a young lady in my youth and then taking up the call to marriage and motherhood here in the states, I had always viewed my husband and myself as missionaries here, right where God had planted us. But I myself had compartmentalized birth to a hospital and had compartmentalized world missions out of it, without even realizing it. Sure I was worshiping the Lord and praying during my births, trying my best to be kind, thankful and appreciative of everything the hospital staff did for me, but I wasn't purposing to be a missionary where I was at or even looking for that opportunity. I am sure as I was worshiping the Lord and experiencing His presence that had made impact on them, but I certainly hadn't been preparing my heart in an intentional way to be a missionary in the hospital when I gave birth.

It's kind of a hard thought to grasp at first, isn't it? Imagine you are in labor and you are called to be a missionary where you are. What does that look like? How on earth can a woman's focus get past her own pain, let alone take advantage of every opportunity to minister for the further advancement of the Kingdom of God?

I think so many times we can get self-consumed that we can't see God's bigger picture unless we sit back and try or unless we ask Him to reveal it to us. There is a huge ministry in the hospital. Many nurses, doctors, midwives and surgeons love Jesus and do what they do because they love Jesus and He has caused them to love people and to heal the sick. If we can go into hospitals with our eyes wide open looking for the opportunities to encourage fellow brothers and sisters in Christ in what they are doing, we can be empowering them to love more. Their duties and the people they serve can suck the joy from them. I have witnessed it myself. It has happened to me. We need to look to encourage them.

On the other hand, there are many doctors, nurses, midwives, and surgeons who do not know Jesus, who may get introduced to Him and who He is by simply watching your testimony play out before their eyes. We need to be alert and aware we are representing Jesus, and we have the power to make a difference. We are called to be missionaries while we are in the hospital, or birth center, or at our home with an unbelieving midwife.

Then there are patients and patients' family members who need Jesus, His love, comfort, and salvation. There are so many opportunities; we just need to ask God to open our eyes so we can see. Make us aware of the pain in people's lives. As we live our lives fully submitted to God while birthing, and we have a host of witnesses (midwives & nurses) who will be ministering to others in birth tomorrow or in a few minutes, they can use what they have learned in witnessing you, to help them, to feed them spiritual nourishment. The opportunity for impact is far greater than just what God wants to do in our lives, dear sister. He wants to do something amazing in others' lives as well.

So for the rest of my pregnancy, I focused and meditated on the concept, the message from the Lord, to be purposeful with the staff and anyone else God had placed in my life throughout this pregnancy, labor, and birth. As I was creating my birth plan, and praying about whom I would choose as my labor partners, I thought about involving my in-laws. In my past three births, my mother had been there with my sister at one. I purposefully invited them, expecting our relationships to grow and the Lord blessed that. But this time it was clear I couldn't expect help from my mom or family because of all my dad was going through. So as I thought on this and prayed about it, it seemed as though the Lord had clearly impressed upon my heart to invite my mother-in-law and sister-in-law.

Under normal circumstances I might not have invited them; after all, birth is a very intimate and spiritual experience. I love my mother-in-law and sister-in-law very much, but it would have been an obvious choice to just invite my mother again. She had already gone through this with me three times, she knew how I labored, what I needed, and I knew I could rely on her spiritual council—this was my mom. Aside from that, I have to admit, the thought of having them at my birth, watching me give birth was a thought I really had to get used to and pray about. Many women have difficult relationships with their "in-laws". Thankfully I can say I am very blessed to have an extremely loving and caring mother-in-law, whom I do have an open and authentic relationship with. But as far as knowing me on a deep spiritual level and experiencing such an intimate experience, I felt like this was uncharted territory. Nonetheless, I had made up my mind to ask them. The Lord had given me the perspective that if I were completely open and vulnerable with them (which you have to be in birth), they would see the real me—all of me—in total dependence on God. This experience would strengthen our relationship unlike anything else. So in faith, and a desire for us to know each other more intimately, I asked them.

As time grew closer, both my mother-in-law as well and my sister-in-law lived with us on and off throughout the summer before Drew was born. I was dilated to a four for about four weeks before he was due, so I felt like a ticking time bomb. I have to share with you what a special time this was to have them living with us. They were such a huge blessing to my husband, my children, and me. Our relationships grew deeper in those six weeks than they had ever been for the six years before. The late night talks, the laughter, the communal living—all of it were just such blessings.

As the due date grew closer, I was tired from juggling between hospital and nursing home visits, prenatal visits, and taking care of three little ones, but having my husband's family there to provide help and stability for my kids was so helpful. Honestly, a part of me wishes it never had to end; life is so much easier with four adults!

The day before Drew was born, my dad was released to come home for the first time in six months. We had a welcome home get together briefly and he and I had a moment I will never forget. As he sat in his chair and I hugged him in full-blown tears, he said, "I am so glad I get to be here to meet my new grandchild, kiddo."

In all those months before Drew's birth, everything in my life had revolved around my dad, without much care to the fact I was pregnant and that was hard for me. Every once in a while my mom would ask how I was feeling, but aside from that all the focus was on Dad. Looking back it is hard for me to admit how selfish my heart was. I had resentment that no-one seemed to be concerned about my health or the stress of sleeping in the hospital for multiple weeks while being pregnant. But isn't that how we all are? Our culture further encourages this selfish thinking during this season in a woman's life.

Then finally one night I let go, of it all, I just simply had built up so many tears, fears, and emotions I wasn't able to express because I was the oldest and I thought I needed to be strong. But that night I let it go, I just cried it out as I walked through our vineyard. I cried, I prayed, I yelled, I praised, and I worshiped. And that night I went into labor free of any stress, resentment, or selfish thoughts, I was ready to embrace my baby in the flesh.

Drew's Birth Story:
A testimony of mission, brokenness, tests, grace, and victory.

Restless and tired, I couldn't sleep. I had been experiencing Braxton-Hicks contractions for weeks, and as I said before, was dilated to a four for a long time. The pressure was taking its toll on my hips. I felt like I was lifting weights around my waist. The next morning, after laboring in and out of the tub all through the night, we ate a good breakfast and headed to the hospital.

Upon arrival, I was calm, as usual. The nurses thought maybe I was having a false alarm simply because of how calm and at peace I was. They had no idea what I had just experienced the last six months, that facing death is much more worthy of panicking over, not facing life! And even in that, I had learned how to not fear death. In all that we had gone through, there was a place where we had to come to peace with death, and because of our faith, we could. I learned God chooses when we leave this earth. He is still in control. So I stood there in peace and joyful anticipation, knowing my dad was alive to meet his grandchild.

Once at the hospital, they checked me in and examined me, and to their amazement I was already at eight centimeters dilated. The nurses rushed out to get the on call midwife. She came in and examined me. I had never met this midwife before; right away she seemed frustrated and non-emotional. Everyone else was so excited we were for sure having a baby today, but she was very stoic. The two nurses on staff helping me were amazing; they were like kindred spirits filing the halls with song as they left our room.

To be honest, in any of my other birthing circumstances, I would have had my husband ask for a different midwife to help us, but I did not because the Lord had impressed upon me the heart to be a missionary and share His love by shining my light through worship and prayer. Based on the fact my first three births were all cut in half in regard to time (four and a half hours, two and a half hours, one and a half hours), we thought that I would have this baby fairly quickly. However, God had His own agenda. As I labored and birth progressed, I experienced dilation every time this particular midwife would examine me. Looking back knowing what I know now about our bodies, I realize it was because I was feeling violated and judged.

You see it was very clear this particular midwife was homosexual, and every time she checked me, she would say, "Well you are making progress slowly, but oh, what are you kidding me? You are de-dilating right now. What are you doing?" She had an angry disposition and spirit about her and clearly did not like me. In fact she even asked Isaac at one point to shut off the worship music so she could focus. Then there was the comment after laboring another ten or eleven hours (at between an eight and ten cm dilated), where she said, "Is this going to be your last baby? Because I have observed women who think they are having their last babies have a harder time with actually letting them come out." It was very obvious she was not comfortable with us and didn't want to be attending our birth either. She scowled at my husband on numerous accounts, as he would ask for things to help me, as if she were annoyed. I am not certain what was really going on with our midwife. It crossed my mind that she might just be having a bad day; but I felt massive judgment from her. I wasn't sure if our faith, worship or our prayer bothered her. Whatever it was I felt compelled to give her grace and just be kind and loving to her.

I was angry with her. I couldn't believe how mean and rude she was. I knew though that I just simply needed to love her. God had placed her there, and He had prepared my heart to be a witness and keep focused on Him. As I labored and I grew more and more weary, I began to lose hope and focus. I looked at my husband, who was by my side the whole time, and I said in short breaths, "I can't do this anymore. I am too tired. I think the baby is stuck. Pray! Just Pray!"

And crying out to God, I said, "I need You!" As we worshipped to "My Utmost for His Highest," I cried. My husband got fully engaged in the intensity of what was going on, and he looked at his mother and said, "When two or more are gathered in prayer, there I am with you, the Lord says. Mom, lay your hands on Angie, we need to pray in the name of Jesus." As they prayed for me, I cried, more than I had cried in a long time. I was empty. Even as they prayed, I was weak. I looked over into the corner of the room and saw my sister-in-law on her knees in the corner of the room. She was either praying or trying to escape the intensity of the reality I was facing. Either way, I felt a connection with both my mother-in-law and my sister-in-law. In those moments of hard work and pleaded to the Lord together, as I had nothing left, I experienced the Holy Spirit fill me up as He "helps us in our weakness. For we do not know what to pray for as we ought, but the Spirit himself intercedes for us with groanings too deep for words," (Romans 8:26).

As the Holy Spirit interceded for me, the bond between my mother-in-law, my sister-in-law, my husband, and me was strengthened. I felt His presence; there was a new energy in the room. The atmosphere of the room was full of love and acceptance, and I felt strong, for just a moment.

When the midwife reentered the room I was determined not to allow her or anyone to steal the Lord's joy or focus on Him from me. Just then, I got on my knees turned around on all fours, looking away from her, my eyes fully locked with my mother-in-law's, while my husband was helping me deliver the baby. I began pushing, but lost hope and strength many times. In that long period of pushing, I felt all kinds of emotions, I was in deep need of Jesus and He was all I could think about. The Lord kept reminding me of 2 Cor. 12:9, "But he said to me, 'My grace is sufficient for you, for my power is made perfect in weakness.' Therefore I will boast all the more gladly about my weaknesses, so that Christ's power may rest on me" (NIV). I cried out to God in my weakness. He was who I sang to as I barely had any breath left. Then, just before our baby was born, I experienced immense fear; I looked straight into my mother-in-laws eyes, intensely focused, she met me there and spoke these words to me, "Yes, you can! God made you to do this." Just then it was like I got a shot in the arm, and I felt Christ's power rest on me. I bore down and I pushed with more might that I had ever felt in my life. And HE was born. All of us crying, my husband said, "It's a BOY!" The nurses down the hall were cheering and singing "Joyful, Joyful We Adore Thee" as it blasted from our room. We were all joyful and in thankful adoration; with the Lord's help, I brought forth a man.

Even in the moments following my birth I could not understand why I was laboring so long. It was a true labor of love. It was hard, but so rewarding. Later though as I thought about it, my suffering and pain might not been about me. I can see that as a believer, if I would have gone into that hospital, had an easy quick birth and had that reputation of being a super-birthing mama none of those nurses or midwives would have gotten to witness what it looks like to truly wait on the Lord for His strength, what it really looks like to worship and praise Him in hard times. Maybe even what my family relationships needed was for me to be empty so we could cry out together, so we could bond and be there laboring together. It made the experience of birth all that much more rewarding.

After my birth, a few of the nurses followed us to the postpartum unit and they came back to see us every day we were there. Neither of them had ever seen a birth like ours before, so they were amazed at what they had witnessed. Nurse Kali had never, in the one hundred and something births she had witnessed, actually witnessed a natural birth. They were in awe of everything about it from how alert the baby was to how quickly I was recovering and how much of a team we were as a married couple and as labor partners with my family. Nurse Kali wrote in Drew's baby journal that "it was beautiful to watch the faith and encouragement of loved ones empowering perseverance."

That night, my mom and dad came to visit me in the hospital. I remember the immense feeling of overwhelming gratitude to God that my dad could walk, with a cane, into that hospital, not as a patient, but as a visitor, to meet his new grandchild. After almost losing him to death on three separate occasions over the course of my pregnancy, finally we had something to rejoice over. New life.

Before they arrived, my husband and I had a very special responsibility—naming our son. We always have a few names on the list, but based upon the birth, what he looked like, the meaning of the name, and what his temperament was like, we had to meet him and get to know him a little. So as I cuddled my sweetest new baby and nursed him, I thought about legacies, I thought about the significance of names. And we chose Drew Titus: Drew meaning wise, courageous warrior and Titus meaning honorable and of the giants. Drew was nine pounds, seven ounces, and to that day my largest baby, with a sixteen and three quarter inch head in diameter. He was of the giants. As we looked into spiritual connotations for the names we chose, this verse especially stood out to me, "But God, who comforts the downcast, comforted us by the coming of Titus," 2 Cor. 7:6. Drew Titus was the only encouraging blessing our family had hope to hang onto for a long season while my father was in the hospital. We were downcast and the Lord renewed our joy with the coming of our son.

This joyful reunion in our room as my parents visited was full of emotion, which the nursing staff witnessed as they carried on their duties of care for me. This led to opportunities for sharing what the Lord had done in my family's life over the past three months. It was a testimony of God's faithfulness.

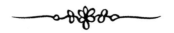

Give God the Plan

Planning, planning, oh how I love it when a plan comes together. Don't you? I think most of us like to have control. Especially in situations like birth, where the unknowns and the what-ifs can create immense anxiety. I have a confession to make: sitting back and giving the reins to someone is really hard for me to do, even giving control to the Lord. I am definitely one who strives for control in most areas of my life. It is a sin for me, one that the Lord is graciously refining me with, and my births have been my refining boot camp. Every day we are alive is a gift from the Lord, and every day brings new opportunities for surrendering our lives completely to Him.

Giving God the control of your life or even your childbirth does not mean we don't prepare or even plan. Nothing in life works like that. Giving God control over our lives inspires us to live more purposefully, more intentional. Being prepared and educated is wise. We have to take personal responsibility for making wise decisions, especially in a life event such as childbirth.

Taking our birth experiences seriously and planning are not going against the concept of giving the Lord control; in fact it is part of the process. Giving Him the control each step of the way, as we get educated and prepare is a spiritual challenge—a challenge to take everything to the Lord in prayer.

There are many beneficial preparatory classes and books to read to prepare you with knowledge and understanding of what to expect while pregnant and giving birth. I highly recommend intentionally pursuing those and learning as much as you can. (*Nesting in Knowledge* is a FREE bonus chapter and book recommendations list available at http://redeemingchildbirth.com)

As Christians who are striving to serve the Lord in all we do, including childbirth, we need to be aware and exercise wisdom in our discernment. Pursue learning about different laboring techniques, and then take what you have learned to the Lord in prayer. Techniques that are neutral (because they are not all neutral in spirituality) are simply just tools. I would encourage you to get educated, do research on the different methods, and then look closely at how each method allows for the involvement of you spiritual convictions. For example, some may have a problem with hypnosis or any other treatment that imposes unconsciousness because they want to be consciously aware so as to pray, worship, and focus on God. As you develop your birth plan and think on these questions, take the questions and your preferences to the Lord. Submit them to Him and purpose to surrender all of your dreams unto the will of the Lord.

There are important things to consider while planning

- Where will your birth take place?
- Are you going to have the baby vaginally or are you planning a caesarean because of health reasons? And WHY? You need to have your convictions as to why.
- How do you plan to manage pain? Water birth? Or epidural? Or neither?
- Who is going to attend your birth? Midwife team, doula, doctor, or hospital midwife?
- What about family and friends? What members of your family are going to attend?

- What technique do I want to learn about and utilize in birth? Who is most familiar with this technique? Then choose to get educated through classes, books, or mentor, midwife, etc.

These are the first key questions to ask as you prepare for this significant day. They are important, not to be assumed that they will be easy to implement when the day comes. It also takes planning to let the Lord have the reins, surrendering all unto Him to rest in His peace. So while you plan, remember to give God your desires, your birth plan. Take them before Him and ask His guidance and protection. Parenting is kind of like planning for your birth and experiencing it. You can hope, dream and plan all you want, but things do not always go exactly as you expected. Some things are harder, some things do come out the way you planned, but in all, God is in control; give Him the control.

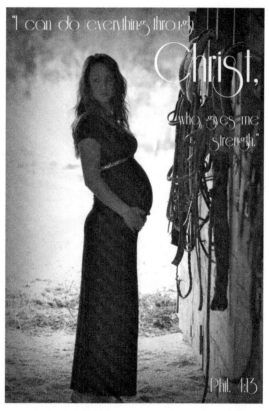

"I can do everything through Christ, who gives me strength."

Phil. 4:13

Things in life get screwed up when we try to take control. Planning is not taking control, it is being wise, not foolish, getting educated, preparing, taking action, and then purposing to submit to whatever the Lord allows for you to experience in your birth experience. Give God the reins and He will be your strength, regardless of what circumstances you may experience.

Choosing Your Birth Attendants

If you have ever run a relay race with a team before, you know that special team bond that only comes from running and sweating together. You have inside jokes from the journey. You are there for one another if there is an injury. You get to know your teammates on a different level. Birth is like a marathon. Who is going to be on your team? You should pray carefully about who God would advise you to choose on this journey, this race, and this intimate experience. Don't forget to invite God! Let Him heal you, let Him have mercy on you, let Him show Himself to you in a new way—a physical, spiritual, emotional way.

> "Therefore, since we are surrounded by a great cloud of witnesses, let us throw off everything that hinders and the sin that so easily entangles, and let us run with perseverance the race marked out for us. Let us fix our eyes on Jesus, the author and perfector of our faith, who for the joy set before him endured the cross, scorning its shame, and sat down at the right hand of the throne of God. Consider him who endured such opposition from sinful men, so that you will not grow weary and lose heart." Hebrews 12:1-4

Choose team members who will encourage you so you do not lose heart or get distracted. Pray for God to reveal who should be at your birth as an advocate, who would make a good encourager, who would be good at keeping your focus on Jesus, and who would be caring and nurturing to your children and husband and their needs (food, etc.) while you are there. God wants to bless you by experiencing the body of Christ in this special way. Let family and friends be His hands and feet by serving you.

"No one knows about the day or hour, not even the angels in heaven, nor the Son, but only the Father. Be on guard! Be alert! You do not know when the time will come." Mark 13:32-33

Surround yourself with encouraging people, a community of saints to keep your focus on the eternal.

Do not be anxious about the timing of your birth! It will happen in God's timing!

Birth is a natural process, but with such spiritual significance. It is not for us to know about the day or the hour. This reality is what most call the mystery of birth. Biblically, there is no mystery. God is the "mystery" miracle worker. He molded that baby from the moment of conception. He has continued to hold that baby in his hands all along the pregnancy. We need to believe He is still holding that baby in His hands through the birthing process, even in regard to all the chemical hormones released in the mother that connect with the baby's neurological system and kick him in gear to cooperate in birth. God created all of those interworkings, and He knows exactly when that baby is going to be born. He is in control. That is what makes each birth such a spiritual experience in and of itself. The Creator God, present with us, in us and working through us, helping us.

A Testimony of God's Sovereign Control

As told by a midwife, Adele, in an interview Feb. 16, 2012.

One of my dear friends and midwife, Adele, shared with me how she was attending one of her granddaughter's births. Once she got there, she realized she didn't have her heart monitor. Since Adele was a seasoned midwife, she always practiced bringing everything legally responsible for a midwife to bring to a birth. As the birth progressed, she really began to get frightened, thinking, "How am I going to hear this baby's heart beat?" As she thought those thoughts, she remembered the Scripture the Lord had given her in the morning, from Job 38-39 where God is interrogating Job, asking him, "Where were you when I laid the earth's foundation. Tell me if you understand." God is making the point about who HE IS! "Do you know when the mountain goats give birth? Do you watch when the doe bears her fawn? Do you know the time they give birth?" God is teaching Job who He is and what He does, where He is at all times, everywhere, in charge of all of life. "They crouch down and bring forth their young; their labor pains are ended. Their young thrive and grow strong in the wilds; they leave and do not return" (Job 39:1-4). Adele described this joyful peace that came over her from recalling how AWE-some God is and who HE is. Just watching her tell the story brought delight and cheery giggles. "Who are we to think we have control over anything by listening to a heart beat?" Although technology is beneficial and extremely useful, we need to remember who is really in control from a spiritual perspective. While using the tools, we need to be careful not to make them idols. "We need to let Him do what He does best. He is ultimately the One doing it anyway." She sat on the side as she watched her daughter give birth to her grandchild. What an emotional moment, when she could have acted panicked, but she remembered her devotional time with the Lord and He spoke peace to her.

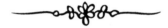

Dare to Dream- God Imparts Dreams and Visions

When Isaac and I went to our first Lamaze class offered at the hospital where we gave birth to our first daughter, I remember doing this exercise where the RN and midwife leading the class had us write down on three cards three different birth scenarios. Plan A was to be our dream birth, what we wished could happen. Plan B was what we think might happen. Plan C was what our nightmare birth would look like. I remember writing out, how I wanted a natural water birth that was short and no perineal tearing, my husband to deliver the baby—all for Plan A. I had high hopes. My Plan B was long labor, exhausted, epidural, needing stitching. My Plan C was an emergency caesarean. The leaders of our pre-birth class went on to direct us to rip up our Plan A cards. And hold onto our other two cards, and try to come to grips with them because most women never get their dream births. Then they went on to teach the statistics for C-sections, epidural rates, percentage of women with tearing and so on. I felt like my dreams were crushed. I was heartbroken over it, but God spoke to me through His word that He is the one who goes before us and plans our steps when we are following His will. So I prayed for God to take my dreams and to give me faith in Him to make them become a reality. I went on to plan for my natural water birth, and the Lord blessed me.

Now, this is not the case with every woman, you know that. But I want to share with you a story of hope. It is ok to dream big, to have a big vision for what you want to experience in birth. The goal is not to follow a plan. The goal is to experience God, and make Him a part of it all the way. If you have done that and it doesn't go the way you planned, that is because God has a different lesson in store for you to learn. You need to surrender to His ways, his good, loving and purposeful ways. All in all, I want to encourage you though, that God wants to be your all-in-all. No matter what laboring method or technique you plan to use while laboring, if your foundational desire is to invite the presence of the Lord to your birth that He may be a part of this intimate event, then God will bless you.

There are other aspects to birth that are wise to plan as well. If you truly desire to give God your birth, invite Him to be the center of your birthing experience, then plan meditative Scriptures, songs for worship, have your labor partners ready to pray with you and intercede for you. Most importantly though, you need to focus *"In his heart a man plans his course, but the Lord determines his steps."* **Prov.16:9** on your walk with Jesus now. Grow in the knowledge and understanding of His Word, learn more about Him, walk with Him, and talk with Him. Then when you are in birth, it will be second nature for you to cry out to Him, to worship Him, pray to Him, and meditate on His word.

Purposefully and prayerfully think about how you want to meet your baby for the first time. Prepare mentally for your delivery day like you would a wedding day. It is the first day you get to visually meet your son or daughter, your only eternal inheritance. Spend some time dreaming, envisioning what your best birth experience could be.

Ultimately, in all the planning you do, go to God in prayer, asking Him to reveal to you His best plan for you! Enjoy the journey of growing in Him, it is a blessing, you don't want to miss.

Planning Your Spiritual Birth Plan

Choosing Your Childbirth Method

Most birthing methods have no spiritual background, but as we have discussed before, some have a new age spin to them. Discerning what is not biblical and omitting it is important as a Christian. However, most methods are simply educational, and train birth coaches and birthing mothers alike in how to birth babies as a team.

Any method can be utilized if one filters out the secular/ new age beliefs and techniques and intentionally chooses to incorporate ones faith in their spiritual birth plan. Certain birthing methods are easier to incorporate one's faith and beliefs though. In my opinion, the Bradley Method complements the biblical model of marriage, teaching the husband and wife how to work together as a team. Water birth is simply a natural way to relieve the pain, anxiety, and physical stress of childbirth while allowing one to embrace the full experience of birth without interventions.

I so want to encourage you younger women just beginning your journey in your childbearing years. There are alternatives that can fit with your spiritual birth plan. You can dream of your "plan A" birth and it can happen. As we have said throughout this book, we are all on our own personal journeys with Christ, so our births will look a bit different. While I may be comfortable in a birthing tub, another sister in Christ might not. My point is we should not judge, but choose to appreciate our differences. There is nothing wrong with our births looking different; it shows our God's awesome creativity in that it reflects the beauty of His creation.

My personal conviction is natural birth is the most gentle and least harmful birth model for both mother and baby, but I do not believe it is an eternal issue. The best decision you can make in regard to choosing your method is to choose what makes you feel most comfortable and still allows you the freedom to personalize those things most important to you and your husband. These stories were merely to stir thought and emotion toward choosing a birthing method that will best meet your end goals as a woman and mother. I believe without hearing stories of the women who have gone before us, we won't be inspired to dream or even know what we should avoid and be on guard against. If we don't know how to dream with realistic hopes, we can miss out on a spiritual blessing of growth in the Lord.

Turning a secular birthing model into a Christ centered method is simple as long as it allows you the freedom to birth how and where you want.

What are some examples of what a Christ-centered birth might look like?

- Praying in birth, independently, with your husband, with your birth attendants, with your children.
- Worshiping in birth through song.
- Experiencing your birth attendants praying together for you and/ or over you.
- The atmosphere of the room focused and centered on Christ.
- You can moan instinctually while having your mind fixed on Him. Being in tune with how God created your body is reflective of appreciating His creation. As you believe and trust He designed you to bring forth life, you may become focused inward and quiet, listening to your body's needs and then acting intuitively, thus bringing glory to God for His design and personally experiencing a growth in trust in Him.
- Intimately leaning on God, experiencing Him give you strength to endure and persevere.
- Staying focused on Jesus, relaxed, remembering to have the joy of the Lord and think about the beautiful baby you are about to hold. Give your anxiety to God; don't be stressed and tense.

- Don't tighten up your mouth, and your body will progress. Tensing up your mouth is counterproductive to labor because your cervix mimics your mouth muscles. If you tighten your jaw in pain, you will actually slow down your labor.

When Christ is the center of your birth, He is the focal point!

It is Him we should cry out to and focus on, not a teddy bear, as our focal point. Make Him the focal point.

When you acknowledge Him and invite Him to be an active comforter, deliverer, creator, Yahweh, the experience is completely different. So different, even I am speechless. Which is the main reason I am writing this book. The only reason actually. God has blessed me and so many other women with amazing stories of experiencing Him in birth. I know when He chose to bless me, it wasn't just for me. It was a gift of knowing Him more fully and deeply that was for all of his daughters. I want that for you. He wants that for you. My sister in the Lord, I want you to experience a deepened faith by embracing the pain that has been predetermined by God for all women in childbirth. Embrace it, do not avoid it.

When you allow yourself to experience the raw, uninhibited pain of childbirth, God can meet you there if you focus on Him and not on the pain. Focus on the image of the cross. Remember the pain He bore for your sins to be washed away, it puts your pain in proper perspective and overwhelms you with thoughts of His grace and love. As you experience this intense pain, think about your baby, and what a gift he/she is from God. Every contraction is making progress toward the moment you will be holding your baby in your arms. Embrace each contraction, use the techniques of breathing that are fantastically helpful in other birthing books, but put your first hope and trust in the Lord. The experience forever changes your spiritual life and impacts your family for generations to come.

This is the foundation of this book—to encourage you to surrender control and your will to the Lord in regard to childbirth. A birth will be centered on Christ if the mother has been focused on Christ and preparing spiritually through her pregnancy. Take all of these things to God in prayer, asking Him to lead you and reveal His plan.

Lord, I pray for my sisters as they pursue learning and deciding which method is best for their marriages and families. I pray they would stay focused on You, Lord. I pray they would look for opportunities to invite You into their experiences as they prepare and plan for this life-changing day. Amen

Part IV

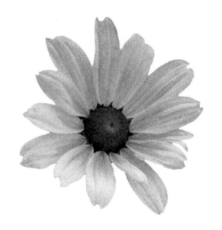

Experiencing His Presence

Inviting the Lord into Our Birth Experience

We've talked thoroughly about the potential for growth in ones relationship with God through the experience of childbirth. Experiencing Him in birth is not something we can accomplish on our own. It is the Lord who blesses us with His presence. I do believe He loves us so deeply that He wants us to desire Him. God wants us to invite Him into every area of our lives, including pregnancy, labor and delivery.

You have a choice to let your pregnancy, labor, and delivery be a catalyst of growth in your life, the tool God uses to refine you. He will refine you either way, but the question is will you learn from it, or ignore the blessing of wisdom and understanding that comes from humbly surrendering all.

The first key is learning to slow down and just be in His presence.

Nothing can quite compare to this intimacy with Christ. When He died on the cross, He took on the pain for our sins. He gave His will to the Father. He committed Himself to the Father even though He foreknew the pain He was about to bear. We can believe God that childbirth is painful, but we can also believe God loves us deeply; so deeply He allowed His one and only Son to be sacrificed for our salvation, for our eternal freedom from the bondage of our sin, that we might be brought back into full unity with our eternal Father and Creator. That bond with our heavenly Father doesn't just happen. We have to take responsibility for submitting our will to Christ, just as He did for His Father on the cross. We have much to learn about sacrifice. The more we focus on being vulnerable in this area of our lives, the more God increases our understanding of His intense love for us. He wants to bless His daughters with all spiritual blessings. When we don't tithe we rob ourselves of God's spiritual blessings and so it is when we avoid experiencing childbirth aware and leaning on Him. Just like tithing is a sacrifice in a sense, we are to do it joyfully. And when we do, the blessing we experience spiritually for being obedient and having acted out our faith is often indescribable. So it is when we step into our childbirth fully surrendered to God's will, whether that be in an emergency situation or a healthy birth plan. Choosing to be fully aware of God working and looking for His goodness and provisions where the spiritual blessing is found.

My aim is not to make anyone feel guilty. But to impress this one thought upon you: why wouldn't a woman want to invite God to be involved and strengthened by His presence in the most emotionally, physically, spiritually, and mentally challenging experience she can experience?

Why do we as Christians go to God purposefully with other requests and not invite Him to be a part of our everyday lives? A woman's birth experience is an intimate one. If you love Jesus, if you depend on Him and lean on Him, why not invite Him to this event? He wants so badly to show you how much He loves you. After giving birth naturally six times now and as an experienced woman, I can clearly articulate what kind of blessing God desires for His daughters. He wants us to embrace Him in our pain. He wants to provide us with supernatural strength when we are at our weakest. He wants to help us through the pain so we can enjoy the first tangible union with our sweet babies. He wants to bless your marriage with mutual respect and with an intense love. He wants you to experience being an intimate team together with Him, the three of you bringing forth man (Gen 3).

Ladies, it comes down to this. What are we created for? What is our purpose? Is it for our selfish desires and our reputations to be great? Is it for furthering our careers or looking like we have the perfect family? Do we exist to glorify ourselves? NO! We are created for a much bigger purpose; we are created to glorify our almighty, omnipotent, and omniscient Creator. We are here to DO what we were designed to do best. We are created for our husbands, to complement them as their other halves. Why? To glorify God! To magnify His name! To shine for Him in this sin-stained, self-indulgent world! We can glorify God in childbirth as Eve did in Genesis 3 when she cried out after birth, "With the HELP of God, I have brought forth man." We, as Christian women, need to birth our babies and bless the Lord. We need to cry out our praises to Him for the magnificent creation He has created within us along with the ability to be blessed and chosen by Him to raise these babies, who have special purposes on earth.

As we allow Him to be a part of our births, we shine for Jesus. We fulfill part of our purposes here on earth. We are blessed to have wombs and blessed to have the opportunity to bring forth man. We need to embrace this awesome gift from God. We need to be overwhelmed with thankfulness. Every time we feel our babies kick, or turn in our wombs, we are bonding with our children. The process of birth is another experience with our child—one of the first. We have the opportunity to introduce them to Jesus when we are pregnant as we pray aloud for them, read the Scriptures to them, and worship through music. Birth is the first time we can truly introduce our children to the power of the Lord.

When you are in labor and feel the temptation to cry out in agony, you can cry to Jesus. You can pray aloud; your baby hears you. If you are the type of person who deals with pain internally, you can withdraw deep inside, intimately with the Lord, and experience His peace and calm serenity for the stirring in your soul. But ladies, we have to purposely do so.

When trials come your way, how do you react? Do you draw near to God? Or do you blame Him? Or are you so distant in your relationship with God that you don't even know where to begin? Jesus desires so deeply for you to pursue Him and Him alone. I believe that is part of the gift of childbirth. He has equipped women since our creation with the gift of anticipating giving birth one day. The gift of this experience is one we should welcome. Allow God to do in your life what He planned to do from the beginning. Take confidence in knowing He designed your body for this amazing calling. Taking confidence in Him means we can give our burdens and fears to Him. We were made to give birth just as many women before us. We were meant to invite God to be a part of the process, following our first mother and example, Eve.

The story of the cross is a love story for us. We can never fully understand the deep love that God has for us, that He would sacrifice His only Son. We cannot fully comprehend the pain Jesus must have felt on that cross, but as women we have been given the gift of having a unique opportunity of experiencing a tiny glimpse of sacrificial pain in childbirth. We as mothers knowingly offer our bodies to go through the pain of childbearing for them to have life. Do not mistake my words we are in NO way even remotely comparable to Jesus. His great sacrifice and the pain He bore for all of our sins, even those mocking Him and wanting Him crucified, was far greater than any pain we could ever imagine. But we can find comfort in the truth that Jesus can empathize with our pain in childbirth. And we should examine our hearts and attitudes against that of what Christ calls us to as believers. Shouldn't we engage the pain in birth following the example He gave us when He endured pain? I believe this is the key element that empowers us to birth differently than the world. If we can turn our eyes to heaven and surrender our will before the Father will in pain, just as Jesus did, then we shine His glory and love to everyone present and we experience the Father's power and strength in those times of need.

We have an opportunity to praise Him and surrender it all to Him. You hear the phrase, "It was painful, but it was worth it." That statement is true. It is wise, but I would like to encourage you to think deeper. Birth is painful, but God is good. The gift of birth is a gift to embrace. We have been given the blessing of feeling the spiritual anointing over our physical bodies when Christ Himself appoints us to the honor of motherhood. Chosen by God to be mothers, we have been given a great honor and privilege. God handpicked us to raise our children (along with our husbands). What a humbling privilege that He would chose us to raise up the next generations.

Preparing spiritually for your birth will benefit you far after your birth. Memorized Scripture that has been meditated on is never a waste. That particular Scripture God gives you for your birth may be meant for more than just your birth experience. You never know when you are going to need to recall the holy Scriptures. And God has a funny way of helping you create memories out of the worship songs you sing while laboring. When I listen to the specific songs my children were born to, it takes me right back to that special time when I was laboring for them with God. I feel His presence all over again and I know just WHO my God is and I remember WHAT He has done for me.

There is nothing that can strengthen your marriage more than working together as a team toward an end goal or a blessing like embracing your baby in your arms.

Pushing while Praying

Prayer: a component of the Christian life that simply is our heart-connection to God, our Savior and Father.

Prayer is expressed through a loving relationship with our Father in heaven. He listens to our prayers simply because He loves us, and we pray because we love Him and want to spend time with Him. We can instantly enter into communication with God, to praise and thank Him for who He is, what He has done, what He is doing, and what He has promised to do. Prayer is one avenue of communication with God where we can share our struggles, needs, wants, fears, trials, and pains, and request His guidance, comfort, provision, and help. God offers His grace and forgiveness to us as we repent and confess our sins openly before Him with a contrite heart in intimate prayer. Praising and thanking the Lord and acknowledging His sacrifices and the pains we have caused Him as our Father in heaven bring us into a more intimate relationship with Him as we grow out of being self-focused in prayer and more aware and thankful for what He has done. In times of mourning and grief, prayer is often acknowledged as the nourishment that causes clarity and perspective as the Lord comforts those who grieve and holds them dear to His heart. Ultimately, prayer is at the core of a personal relationship with God because it is the communication between you and Him. Honest (transparent/ giving) communication is what relationships thrive on. Without it, a relationship would cease to exist on a personal level.

There are those who know about God and those who know God. Prayer is the evidence of the depth of both.

I think it is safe to say that in our culture, being busy is idolized as significant while being disciplined in prayer is not, and those who embrace prayer battle everyday to be countercultural and purposeful in finding time to be still and talk with God. Our souls cry out for spiritual connection to our heavenly Father, but we deprive ourselves by getting distracted by things of less value, things that are not eternal. This is especially true in preparing for birth and motherhood when it is easy to get distracted with things of lesser eternal value and importance than prayer.

Prayer is not something we should simply do routinely at meals, at bedtime, in church, or only after we have gotten everything else done. Prayer is something we need to prioritize in our lives. I am not talking about having to pencil God into your schedule, although for some that may be necessary. I am talking about living as if God really is our first priority in life. I have to admit here, this is all very convicting to me as well. I have failed in the area of disciplined alone time in prayer during busy seasons with little babies and toddlers, but I was a better mom in those days when I had my time with Him. So why do I feel so compelled to include talking about prayer in a book on childbirth? Because it was my personal prayer testimony that God used in my pregnancies and births to increase my faith and draw me into a more intimate relationship with Him and those closest to me. I have been ever changed as a woman because of the depth of His teaching, nurturing, and provision for me during these experiences.

You are probably thinking, oh yes, it makes sense that prayer should be covered in a book titled *Redeeming Childbirth*. Clearly, after reading this book, I am sure you will be more aware of the need for prayer. We, as a church, need to pray for our world, our churches, our view of children and birth, and our fears and the lies we have believed. Pregnancy and childbirth offer many opportunities for mothers-to-be to lean on the Lord through prayer and experience His presence in what can be one of the most challenging but sanctifying (growing) life transitions we encounter. It is foundational that as we pursue spiritual growth in the Lord we develop our relationship with Jesus through prayer, worship and meditative study of His word. As followers of Christ, we are so blessed that He allows us to come into His presence through prayer. He meets us personally and collectively as a church body, and promises, "For where two or three are gathered in my name, there am I among them," (Matthew 18:20).

Why is prayer so essential in Redeeming Childbirth?

1.) No woman can fully surrender her birth under the headship of Christ, for Him to redeem it, if she has not surrendered her life to Jesus Christ in repentant prayer. As you seek God and strive to live for Him, prayer is that lifeline of intimacy. It is because of His great love for us all that He has made a way for us to meet with Him. God didn't have to . . . but He wanted to. He wants to lead our hearts and create in us passions that are in alignment with His will for our lives. He wants to know us deeply and intimately. He wants us to lean on Him for every decision in life. The more connected we are to God in prayer the more we will desire to live fully submitted to Him and His plan for our lives. God so deeply wants us to know the abundance of His love. He can provide all we need and more than we could hope for in life situations that, according to the world, are to be feared or dreaded. In thankfulness, we should be overwhelmed with His loving kindness and desire to glorify His name for what He has done. When you experience God in such an intimate way, like in labor and birth, you can't help but glorify Him. Ronnie Floyd writes, "Through prayer, God establishes a trust relationship with you and me, our faith is enlarged when God's activity becomes evident in our lives."[20]

2.) Prayer has the power to influence circumstances, if you are praying in His will. "This is the confidence we have in approaching God: that if we ask anything according to his will, he hears us. And if we know that he hears us—whatever we ask—we know that we have what we asked of him," (1 John 5:14-15, NIV). The key is in praying for His desires for your life and the lives of others. Acknowledging that sanctification is a refining process by which we grow through life's circumstances helps us to understand the purposes behind why we are allowed to experience certain trials in life. Praying in His will does not always mean we are praying for an easy life; in fact, quite the contrary. If we desire to grow, we can count on the fact that we will experience hard times. Childbirth is not easy, it is hard, but it is good. It is refining. Parenthood is fun and life fulfilling but sometimes it is also hard but good in that we grow much from being parents.

God says in his Word, "Ask and it will be given to you; seek and you will find; knock and the door will be opened to you," (Matthew 7:7, NIV).

3.) Prayerlessness means you are either depending on yourself (Genesis 4:25-26), you don't have the conviction that God is worthy of your time, or you just don't know how to pray. I realized that by not praying, I was subconsciously and arrogantly acting in my own sufficiency and not recognizing my deep need to call upon the Lord and follow His will. I was relying on my own wisdom to make the right decisions and my strength to have control over circumstances. Childbirth and parenthood will be a rude awakening for the individual who lives in prayerlessness. Motherhood is truly a labor of love that lasts as long as life. I grieve for the woman who carries that burden on her own.

God Wants Us to Cry Out to Him

When a woman cries out to God in prayer in labor and birth, she invites Him to be present there.

From the time a mother finds out she is pregnant, she begins dreaming about who her child will become. What will he/she look like? What type of personality will he/she have? What will God's path be for his/her life? She begins dealing with fears about the health of her baby, the birth process, her ability to be a good mother, and so many more. Some women experience complicated pregnancies, morning sickness, bed rest, preterm labor symptoms, and more severe emergencies. For these women, learning how to trust and lean on God has a different meaning than it does for those who have full-term healthy and predictable pregnancies. Women with difficult pregnancies who rely on Him experience an extra-ordinary growth process and sanctification through their many moments of reaching out to God and wrestling with Him, crying "Why God? Why Me? Why my baby?" As Richard Foster puts it in *Prayer*, "when we pray, genuinely pray, the real condition of our heart is revealed. This is as it should be. This is when God truly begins to work with us. The adventure is just beginning. . . . We pace the floor with God, telling him of our hurt and our pain and our disappointment . . . frustration and tears and anger are also the language of Simple Prayer. We invite God to walk with us as we grieve the loss of our dream . . . we speak frankly and honestly with God about what is happening and ask him to help us see the hurt behind the emotion. We should feel perfectly free to complain to God, or argue with God or yell at God."[21]

There are many examples of prophets and men of faith who questioned, defied, wrestled or even shouted at God in Scripture (see Jer. 20:7; Genesis 32; and the book of Jonah). Again quoting from Foster, "C.S. Lewis counsels us to 'lay before Him what is in us, not what ought to be in us.' We must never believe the lie that says that the details of our lives are not the proper content of prayer."[22]

Once in labor, the anticipation and anxiety of what is to come is clearly a time when focusing on the Lord is more than appropriate. When you are in childbirth, there are many intense moments when you have to reach deep within yourself without focusing on yourself and instead focusing on God. Times like these are the perfect opportunity to call on the Lord and set your eyes on things above, on Jesus, rather than your own pain or fear. Psalm 91:14-15 says, "The Lord says, 'I will rescue those who love me, I will protect those who trust in my name. When they call on me, I will answer.'"

Inviting God to Redeem Your Childbirth through Prayer

Please do not assume that because you read this book and it sounds like a great idea to pray through birth that you will. We are all on our own spiritual paths, and while I am still learning much about prayer, many who read this are much more mature than I am in this area. On the other hand, there may be younger Christians reading this who have no idea how to even begin praying. The purpose of this chapter is to equip some with tools on how to prepare to pray in birth. For some, it will simply encourage you to incorporate more of God in childbirth and relationships. For others, it will whet your palette for deeper faith and ignite a personal prayer relationship between God and one of His daughters.

Prayer is such a broad and deep topic, but the concept is simple—it is communication with God. It is as simple as just talking with Him about anything and everything, and as reflective as meditating on His sacrifice on the cross and being overwhelmed to mourning and tears in true knowledge and understanding of what He suffered on our behalf. Prayer can be filled with praise and worship by focusing on His attributes and acknowledging who He is. It invites God to be an active part of your life. To pray takes humility; to see ourselves through a realistic lens, leading us to understand our need for God. When you come to the Lord, humbled before Him, aware of His attributes and of your sin and inability to do anything holy or righteous apart from Him, you recognize your need for Him. In childbirth, in order for women to gracefully embrace the whole experience of birth, we need to rely on God and His strength. We cannot redeem our own childbirth; Jesus is the one and only redeemer.

Pray with me

Lord Jesus, I believe in You and Your great power. I believe You have the power to heal, to do miracles, and to open and close wombs as You please. You created my body in the secret place and designed me to bring forth life. You have blessed me with this gift of life You are forming in my womb and I am so grateful. Thank You, Lord, for blessing our family with an eternal heritage. Thank You for always being here to hear me, even when I sin against You and those I love. Please create in me a clean and teachable heart. Help me to desire Your will for my life and to do my part in pursuing it. Thank You for giving me a purpose in life. I surrender my life to You. Use me to make a difference in this world for the advancement of Your kingdom. Help me not to simply settle for what I can do in life, but experience what You can do. Help me keep my mind stayed on You so that my heart will continue to yearn for more of You. Jesus, please be with me when I go into labor. Help me to focus on You and be sensitive to Your Spirit. If there is a nurse or a family member who needs to know You and they are at my birth, help me to be so focused on serving You that I can shine Your light even in the midst of contractions. Please protect my baby and me. Give me strength and help me not to fear the unknown. I desire so badly to have a natural birth, but everyone around me doubts if I will be strong enough. Lord, I know I am not, but I believe You are, and with Your help, I can do all things. Lord, please use this experience to strengthen my marriage. May I be a good example to my daughters of how to worship You and lean on You for strength in childbirth. I pray I don't scare them from having children, Lord. May it teach my children what it means to surrender all to You and may they be drawn into an authentic relationship with you because of witnessing and experiencing Your presence. Redeem my childbirth, Lord; have Your will be done in me. May I shine Your light to all who see and hear my prayers *and may You be glorified through me. Jesus, You are my strength when I am weak, You are my all-in-all. I am nothing without You but can do anything with You. And I thank you that you are always with me. My desire is to hear You say, "Well done my good and faithful servant." May I bring joy to You, Lord, as I do Your will. Amen.*

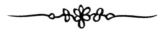

So How Do We Invite God to Redeem Our Childbirth?

We can invite the Lord to redeem our childbirth through prayer and by surrendering our dreams, desires, and hopes for our birth to Him, giving Him complete control. Just as we surrender our lives to the Lord and recommit to Him daily in prayer, we also can commit this experience to Him in prayer.

But how do we experience His strength in the midst of contractions, when one is tempted to let fear overcome? God bestows strength; it is not something we can will, although we need to do our part by focusing on Him in prayer. As we continue to pray through birth, relying on God to keep our minds stayed on Him, we experience His presence.

Staying focused on the Lord and recommitting to Him throughout birth is not easy. As humans we are constantly distracted and tempted to try to take control of our lives and circumstances. In hospitals, one of the biggest distractions is the potential pressure to utilize interventions and submit control to a doctor. In certain circumstances or emergencies, this is extremely appropriate. However, in healthy births, interventions are usually used for convenience, expediency, and to avoid childbirth pain. Why do I bring up drugs? Is it eternal if a woman uses drugs? No, but my question is aimed at the motives and heart-attitudes behind why a woman would chose pain medications? And that is not something we can judge for anyone else. It is personal between a woman and her God what her attitudes and motives are and why they are what they are.

In natural birth, doctors and labor partners may ask you if you want to use interventions for a variety of reasons. Some doctors really do have your best interest in mind . . . or at least have pure intentions. They don't know the real reasons you have chosen to pursue natural birth and that being offered drugs is frustrating for you. In those cases simply be kind in how you speak with them, but use it as an opportunity to witness in love or share with them what you are learning and trying to incorporate in your birth (faith) experience. This is where having dedicated your birth to the Lord throughout the pregnancy is important. Our lives are in the Lord's hands and so are the lives of our babies. No matter how much control we try to take, He is the author of life. If we devote ourselves to seeking His will for our lives and our birth experiences, we can stand with the confidence of the Lord either way. If an emergency does occur, having an intimate relationship with the Lord is crucial in walking through those realities. If you are experiencing normal birth pains, having an intimate relationship with Jesus allows you to experience His presence; leaning on Him as He empowers you with supernatural focus and strength of will to keep on keepin' on. A relationship with God is developed similarly to other relationships—over time and authentic communication.

Who do you go to with your concerns, troubles, wants, and needs? When life is going good or great even, to whom do you give the glory? Do you go to your husband first, a good friend, your mom, or do you go to God? Do you take the glory that belongs to the Lord simply by forgetting to thank Him? It isn't bad to go to others with your needs, especially if you are taking them the requests to be praying with you, but you should first go to God. Prayer is our heart connection with God. As spiritual beings, God made us to desire that spiritual heart connection. I find that when I don't seek God but instead desire to have alone time with my husband or a ladies night out for conversation, I am just attempting to fill a void that only God can fill. I am not saying those nights out are bad. Quite the contrary, I am a big fan of date nights and connecting with like-minded kindred spirits. However, we should not be seeking those things first when God is the only one who can fill us up. When we do not get filled up, we have less to give to others and oftentimes it also drastically changes our heart attitudes. Our heart attitudes are a fruit of the Spirit, which is molding us as we are abiding in Him. The key is abiding in Him, allowing our heart attitudes to be malleable and teachable as we walk through life's experiences, trials, joys, and circumstances. It is not natural for us to embrace the concept of letting God transform us and mold us to be more like His Son. We need a heart that is soft to His ways and His will in order for Him to sanctify us. Our hearts don't become soft on their own; it is through intimacy with God in prayer that the Holy Spirit is invited to change our hearts. Prayer cultivates transformation of the heart.

Just as the depth of your relationship with God can be revealed through prayer, so can your faith and depth of relationship be revealed through how you handle the hard moments in birth. When we humans are in pain, we have numerous response options. We can curse God and rely on ourselves and our own strength, or pray and cry out to God. We can faithfully believe in His goodness and simply trust in His peace and focus on Him. We all deal with circumstances in life differently. But the truth is that the depth of what is in our hearts is revealed and God gives us examples of how we should respond to life's circumstances. In Job 1:20-22, after Job had heard from the messenger that all of his family had been killed and everything was taken away, his response was to worship and praise God. In his mourning, He cried out to God, "At this, Job got up and tore his robe and shaved his head. Then he fell to the ground in worship and said: 'Naked I came from my mother's womb, and naked I will depart. The Lord gave and the Lord has taken away; may the name of the Lord be praised.' In all this, Job did not sin by charging God with wrongdoing," (NIV).

So how do you prepare for the unknown? Not in fear, that's for sure. No, the best advice I feel compelled to give and the foundation of this book is to prepare your soul, your relationship with God. Spend this season in your life focused on Jesus, learning about Him, studying the Word, and developing a deeper love relationship with Him through prayer. Develop the disciplines of the Christian faith now; finding the time won't get easier after you have children. Create the habit of putting God first in all your relationships. Make God number one! None of us know what the future holds, but we are given direction for what to do today: to worship, praise, thank Him, know about Him through studying the Bible, know Him through prayer, serve Him, obey Him, and surrender our lives under His headship. When we do what we are commanded to do, loving the Lord with our whole hearts, soul, mind, and strength, we are more prepared for life.

Prayer is like a muscle in your relationship with God; the more it is exercised the stronger your relationship with God will be. It is the same with knowing anyone else intimately, the more time and honest communication is invested, the deeper the relationship. A key to a truly deep relationship with anyone is when you can be uninhibited and transparent with one another and you can share with them the depth of your relationship with God without fearing what they will think. Let's build those relationships, ladies, so we can encourage one another toward good works. Then our relationships can be catalysts toward a stronger relationship with God as we serve Him together and experience His presence through prayer and worship. May God use us, our relationships, our testimonies, and our birth stories to glorify the Lord and help expand His kingdom.

Prayer is not a formula, but we do need to develop the discipline!

When preparing for birth and developing a closer relationship with God through prayer, you will find there is no formula for praying. Jesus did give us many examples of prayers all throughout the scriptures: the Lord's Prayer found in Matthew 6:9-13, the prayer in the garden of Gethsemane in Luke 26:39-46, the Psalms, Job's cry (Job 1:20-22), the Prayer of Jabez in 1 Chronicles 4:10, and so many more. Knowing God empowers us to experience His true holy joy when we receive our precious babies in our arms. You know that feeling of holding a baby after having labored. You treasure the gift of your baby more because of the journey of pregnancy, labor, and birth. I have met women who have struggled with infertility, who after years of trying to become pregnant finally have babies and their perspectives are very different than most in our culture. These women genuinely value the true gift of life so much more because of their challenge in receiving the gift in the first place. It is also very similar for adoptive mothers who for years tried and prayed for children. These women have experienced a different but similar sanctifying pain. Their love and perspective for children is one part of what has redeemed their pain and sorrow in not being able to go through childbirth. They too have experienced sorrow like a mother in childbirth, aching for their eternal inheritance, their gift to be given by the Giver of life.

If we didn't experience any challenges in the process of pregnancy, labor, or birth, I dare to wonder how we would value children today. It is these challenges that strengthen how we value children and gratefulness for them. It is the challenge we overcome in birth that breeds such joy in our souls as we enjoy our babies. I always grieve for my sweet sisters who don't have the joy of experiencing this elation. I grieve because there is scientific evidence that proves the correspondence between hormonal/emotional affects and usage of interventions. I say this to warn you of the truth, but also to comfort those who may have struggled in the past with transitioning to motherhood. It may not have been anything about your body, it might have been the medication. And if so, you have hope for future births that it doesn't need to be the same story. God can redeem your childbirth.

Your baby symbolizes many things, including the victory you personally experienced as you endured and persevered. Joy is so apparent in women who have given birth and have surrendered to the Lord because their identities, which were founded on Christ, have been strengthened in Him from having experienced His presence and empowering strength in childbirth.

For those who are new to Christianity or just beginning a journey of knowing God intimately, I pray you are encouraged to seek Him personally. Thankfully, there is no wrong way to pray. Since prayer is such an essential element to a personal relationship with Christ, He has provided us with many examples of how to pray.

We can pray alone or in community with others

- You can pray quietly in your own room, "But when you pray, go into your room, close the door and pray to your Father, who is unseen. Then your Father, who sees what is done in secret, will reward you," (Matthew 6:6, NIV).

- We can pray collectively, "Again, I tell you that if two of you on earth agree about anything you ask for, it will be done for you by my Father in heaven," (Matthew 18:19, NIV). Praying together with the body of Christ strengthens and edifies the church.

Prayer Is Personal

Our relationships with God are intimate and personal and therefore are unique and will look different for each of us. One truth is that we all need to practice the spiritual discipline of prayer. It is the lifeline of our relationship with our Father, Savior, Counselor, and Friend. Keep it real, God is not concerned with your vocabulary, He wants your attention and heart.

- **Conversational Prayer** doesn't have to be eloquent or knowledge-based. Simple prayer, as taught about in Richard Foster's book *Prayer*, is simply:
  - Sharing your heart, your feelings, your hurts, wants, desires and needs.

- Crying out to God, wrestling with Him about life's trials and challenges.
- Thanking Him for His help and provision.

When you are in labor and your contractions are strong and you feel like you can barely speak, let alone pray, use simple prayer. Just talk to God; be honest before Him and if you cannot verbalize what you need then ask your husband and those there with you to pray on your behalf.

- **Pray Scripture.** Prayers can and should be inspired by the Bible. When reading the Word of God it has the power to convict, to equip, to teach, and to empower vision. When you pray, incorporating scripture literally ensures you to be praying the will of God. It promises to give whatever we ask if it is in His will.

- **Pray in the name of Jesus.** It is the power of His name that is our gateway to God:

- **Pray Specifically.** When you study scripture, the requests people asked of Jesus when He walked the earth were very specific. His mother asked Him to turn water into wine. People asked for specific healing. Why would we communicate any different today? When my children ask me for something, they are usually very specific. If they are not they usually do not get what they are expecting. We should not be afraid to ask God specifically to meet our needs or to grant us the desires of our heart (when they are in His will).

- **Pray Under the Leadership of the Holy Spirit.**
  Do you pray through an agenda? Do you pray only habitually, routinely at meals, bedtime, when in an emergency or in times of need? Ronnie Floyd writes, "When you pray under the leadership of the Holy Spirit you cannot be in a hurry."[23]

Praying under the leadership of the Holy Spirit can be praying frequently throughout the day whenever the Lord prompts you.

"I am the gate; whoever enters through me will be saved." John 10:9, NIV

However, intentional prayer happens when you give God your undivided attention either for two minutes or two hours.

How can you begin to pray according to the leadership of the Holy Spirit?

You begin with moments of not saying anything. Meditate on the things of God. I would encourage you to begin praying something

"Until now you have asked nothing in my name. Ask, and you will receive, that your joy may be full." John 16:24

like, "Lord, I come to you in the name of Jesus Christ today. I do not want to have a moment of vain repetition that will not please you but I want you to show me what to pray for right now."[24]

When you pray under the leadership of the Holy Spirit, you will receive His power when you pray and then mighty things begin to happen. Praying under the leadership of the Holy Spirit can only happen when you are not focused on yourself. You need to be completely attentive to the Spirit and His promptings.

"Therefore God exalted him to the highest place and gave him the name that is above every name, that at the name of Jesus every knee should bow, in heaven and on earth and under the earth, and every tongue acknowledge that Jesus Christ is Lord, to the glory of God the Father." Phil 2:9-11, NIV

Begin now

Use this time of pregnancy to seek God, to seek His will, instruction, and wisdom.

As the due date approaches and excitement grows, there are mixed feelings (and hormones) of being blessed with a child and feeling overwhelmed with the reality of how your life is about to change. Pregnancy is a season in a woman's life when she has the opportunity to grow in faith as she leans on her Lord. Prayer is the key ingredient to gracefully embrace His miracle in your life. When you connect with God in prayer, you have the opportunity to surrender your labor and birth unto Him, asking Him to redeem your birth. As I mentioned earlier, this will look different for every woman.

*If some of the words mentioned in this chapter are unfamiliar to you, please don't be discouraged, but rather let it motivate you to learn and study. Our relationships with God never hit a place of accomplishment or having arrived. We are all sinful and in need of growth and sanctification. We are all in this together. Let's be united in spirit, encouraging, equipping, and inspiring one another toward good works, knowing about Him and knowing Him more intimately. Prayer is such a broad topic, and this book is not about prayer, but I do want to equip you, my friends and fellow mothers, by hopefully planting a seed of thirst and hunger within you for a deep heart connection with God through prayer. There are many wise books on prayer so go and pick out a few. Invest time deepening your relationship with the Lord now before your baby is born. It will be a foundation for you to grow on through life. Motherhood is a labor of love; it does not end after birth. When you begin this journey of parenthood and have experienced Him in such an intimate way, you are empowered to "continue in faith and love and holiness, with self control," (1 Timothy 2:15). Your faith and relationship with the Lord can be strengthened through the experience of childbirth as you rely on Him and experience Him giving you strength and having mercy on you as He delivers you.

Your birth testimony can become a milestone worthy of an altar of remembrance in your faith journey.

When Two or More Are Gathered

One way God can do His redeeming work is by working in the lives of those involved in your labor and birth. As you make yourself vulnerable to the Lord's work by intentionally involving family members, allowing them to be present in your birth and praying with you, God begins doing a redeeming work through your childbirth. Families are strengthened in many ways: marriages are built up as a team, mothers and daughters are brought to unity, sisters mentor sisters and minister to one another, and children are able to witness God's presence and see Him at work. When the body of Christ is allowed to be God's hands and feet then He is not only present in your birth, but taking part in something He is usually alienated from, and shines His glory all through it.

A Like-Minded Community of Saints

The blessing of a community of saints, praying for you while you are in birth goes beyond expression. I cannot urge to you enough the incredible blessing it is to have godly women in your life who are lifting you up in prayer whether you are struggling in pregnancy, in labor, delivery, postpartum recovery, and even just as you are parenting. I have personally been so blessed with countless women who have a deep love and respect for the power of prayer. When you go from being depressed from vomiting to having joy in your heart while the circumstances of your condition haven't changed, you know you are experiencing the power of prayer in your life. This is such a blessing while in birth, but is not something many women focus on preparing for. I urge you sisters in the Lord, to spend time praying and asking God for other Christian sisters who would be willing and disciplined to commit as your prayer partners during your pregnancy and birth (either physically at the birth or not), and while you are adjusting and recovering from childbirth. Finding a community of women who can lift you, your family, and your baby up in prayer is a prerequisite to experiencing a consistent prayer support source for you during your birth process.

Another suggestion that is extremely beneficial in the actual birthing experience is choosing labor partners who you are developing relationships of prayer with, so when you are in those moments when you need others praying over/for you, they can sense it and take action, interceding on your behalf. If you or your labor partners are not comfortable praying in front of one another in normal circumstances, chances are they are not going to feel comfortable praying in front of other people—especially nurses and others. These relationships don't just happen. It takes being intentional about growing the relationship to a level of transparency and a deep love for carrying one another's burdens, and a mutual belief that God is the only one who can remedy a trial or offer such gifts as strength, supernatural power, and patience. Purposefully choosing friendships and relationships and encouraging them to be God-focused are the first steps. What I am talking about here is authentic friendships that are deeper than an acquaintance and resemble a sisterhood in Christ, which is what being a part of the body truly is. These are the friendships that are typically referred to as kindred spirits. After seeking out these real friendships that are Christ-centered, then you can openly discuss your prayer objectives, your accountability fears, and your desires for your birth experience and a commitment for support. Developing these friendships is key to having a community of saints supporting you throughout life and who you can support as well. I believe this is the true picture of the Body of Christ; coming together purposefully, praying together in a time of need. After praying for God to make clear who will be your birth attendants, it is important to be clear in your communication with your labor partners. Share with them your desires and plan for your birth and guide them in how they can specifically minister to your needs. Learning about intercessory prayer together and their role in inviting the Lord to be present and active is also an opportunity for growth personally and collectively as the body of Christ.

The point is that it takes effort, discipline, and a desire to intentionally build a community of sisters in the Lord who can walk through life with you, and you with them, ministering to one another. Relationships take time. There are a million distractions when you get together with a sister in the Lord. You may fully intend on praying together, but it takes discipline to actually spend the time doing it. The desire to seek out friends comes from understanding the importance of being a part of a community that is there for one another through good times and bad. Not everyone in this life is ready for a transparent relationship, nor do many know what that even looks like. It takes desire to keep trying with different people, until you find those like-minded souls who have their identities in the Lord and can rejoice with you when you rejoice and who can stand strong and speak the hard truth when it is necessary as well.

The Power of a Praying Husband in Birth

Just as you cannot assume that your labor partners are going to be comfortable praying for your childbirth if you have not prayed with them regularly before your birth, the same applies to your husband. A woman cannot expect her husband to be a prayer warrior in her labor and birth if they have not prayed together at home. If a man is not comfortable or practiced/disciplined at prayer in front of you, in the privacy of your own room, then you cannot expect him to be comfortable and eager to be praying aloud over you in front of a hospital staff, a mother-in-law, or others who happen to be present during the birth. Prayer is an intimate conversation, and when a couple prays together, they are ushered into an intimacy with God together. As you both share your hearts aloud before God, you are sharing your fears and concerns in front of one another as well as thanking God for the things He is teaching you. Many of these things go unsaid in marriage, but when you take the time to pray together, you see another side of your spouse's heart. Knowing what is going on in his heart deepens the marriage relationship, but doing so in the presence of the Lord adds another spiritual element that cannot be derived. If you have not experienced this intimacy with your spouse before it does not mean that you shouldn't expect him to pray with or for you during labor and birth. But it does mean you need to communicate with your husband about it and begin practicing the discipline of praying together regularly, if you don't do that already. In addition, you need to fully communicate your spiritual desires and plans for your birth with your husband.

Our husbands were designed by God to be our protectors! Let your husband be who God made him to be for you! Practice having him lead you in husband-coached birth exercises. Or do a husband-coached birth education class together. Even reading a book together to help him be more prepared for what to expect and to get him as involved as possible is going to improve your intimacy in the birth. The most important thing you can do is to be clear and share your expectations for the day you give birth. Communicate!

The Strength of Intimate Mother, Daughter, and Sister Relationships

Mother, daughter, and sister relationships are examples of relationships that should be purposefully developed to be your strongest advocates in birth and life. The unconditional love and depth of desire for your best interests, especially when centered on Christ, can prove to be very powerful in childbirth. God has blessed us with these unique relationships for many reasons. We can shine His light together as a body or team whose members deeply love and care for one another and petition for one another's best interests through intercessory prayer. Developing these relationships does not happen overnight. It takes patience, earnest intent, and time; but once developed, these relationships prove to be a huge blessing that cannot compare to any other.

Your childbirth is a fantastic opportunity to engage your sisters and mothers in a way that makes them feel appreciated and honored for being such an important part of your life. This intimate experience allows you to share your heart and love for the Lord with those in your family, creating a camaraderie that cannot be created any other way. My births are some of the most intimate spiritual experiences in my life. To be able to share that with my sister and sister-in-law was a privilege.

Having your mother at your birth helps to transition your relationship naturally and in a healthy way. All mothers struggle with allowing their babies to grow up in one regard or another. When a mother is allowed to be there for her daughter's birth, I believe it not only strengthens their relationship, but also brings the new grandmother to a conscious realization that her daughter is growing up or has grown up. God designed mothers to nurture, that deep and God-instituted nature does not disappear the day her daughter is married. I believe this innate desire to care for your children is never extinguished.

When we, as daughters, allow our mothers the God-given right to nurture and care for us in birth, they feel fulfilled. It is a rite of passage, like a father walking his daughter down the aisle. As your mother watches you lean on God, worshiping Him and allowing Him to redeem your birth, her respect for you as a mother will grow immensely. And as she watches your husband care for you as your primary birthing coach, her faith in your marriage and in his care for you as a protector and head of the household will also grow. She will have to sit back and wait for you and your husband to involve her, which is good practice for her as a grandmother-to-be. Childbirth can also serve as a boot camp for grandmothers as they learn their position of authority in your family. The experience teaches them to rely on God in a new way as they pray for you and watch you give birth, but are helpless in taking your pain away. And because our mothers have given birth to us, there is an unspoken bond and camaraderie that is formed as they watch you give birth and become a mother. There also is a simultaneous gain of respect that takes place: in your mother for you as a woman and a new mother, and in you for your mother who went through this same sanctifying experience for you.

Discipling Your Children in Prayer through the Season of Childbirth

Praying with your children through life's circumstances and experiences is part of "training up a child in the way he should go," (Prov. 22:6, NIV).

One way your children can participate in their baby brother or sister's birth process is by including them when you are praying for your unborn child. The more you involve your children in praying together for their new sibling the more their hearts will grow and the better they'll be prepared for the adjustment of a new addition to the family. Inviting them to pray often is also one way to disciple (or mentor) up your children in the Christian faith. If you choose to have your children present at your birth, they will not only witness a baby being born, but also be mentored through modeling how to pray and worship the Lord in all circumstances. They will no longer view birth as this mysterious life-event that is compartmentalized to the hospital, but as a natural life-event that can incorporate God anywhere, in any way, and with anyone present. However, involving your children this intimately is not for every family, marriage, or child. It truly takes knowing if your children are mature enough and whether you are comfortable with them witnessing it. More importantly, it takes prayer and asking God what His will is for your whole family with regard to this decision and being open to being asked by God to step out of culturally influenced comfort zones. Receiving another child from the Lord impacts everyone in the family. I would encourage you to seek His wisdom in determining how involved you want your children to be in this life process because the blessings that come from it cannot be compared to any other.

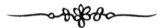

Let's pray

Lord, I know I have not even begun to cover the tip of the iceberg with regard to what You can do in the labor and birth of a child. Please accept this attempt to teach and equip my sisters in surrendering their births to You for the bigger picture: Your vision and Your will for their lives. Thank You for what You have taught me as I have written this word. May it be pleasing to You, O God. Amen.

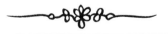

Ideas to Implement:

1) Start a prayer journal.

2) Create a schedule or plan a specific time to pray every day that is not going to be rushed (mine is while in the shower).

3) Talk to God every day, all day, and throughout the day. Remember, He is always with you. He truly is your best friend and doesn't have to be formal.

4) Pray with your husband and if you don't already, talk with him about it. I have found praying with my husband helps me know what is really in his heart. Then you will be more inclined to continue praying for his requests until you pray together again. Strong marriages pray together.

5) Think about and pray about who God may want you to invite to your birth (mother, mother-in-law, sister, friend, daughter, etc.).

6) Begin praying with your children now if you plan is to have them involved in your birth somehow. It helps to prepare their hearts for the experience and opens up lines of communication. You will get to hear their fears and then can talk about them. Also, this provides an opportunity for you to disciple your children in prayer and in preparation for having a baby—two invaluable experiences in the Christian faith.

7) Choose one prayer method that you may not be as familiar with (prayer that acknowledges the attributes of God) and begin to implement it to challenge yourself.

8) If you haven't ever read a book on prayer, I would highly suggest reading one.

Crowning Him in Worship

What words, thoughts, and meditations of the heart are pleasing to God? Words, thoughts, and meditations that are a reflection of a conviction that He alone is to be praised, He alone is to be worshiped, He alone is thanked, adored, loved, obeyed, and glorified.

When I first starting thinking about how to share with other women the concept of worshiping God in childbirth, I honestly couldn't think of a simple way to express how spiritually enriching it is. When you approach your child's birth in faith,

> *"Let the words of my mouth and the meditation of my heart be pleasing to you, O Lord, my rock and my redeemer."*
> **Psalm 19:14, NLT**

relying on God, and focusing on Him through worship, it can impact your spiritual life forever. Worship is an essential ingredient in experiencing His presence in any event in life, including childbirth.

The combination of approaching birth as an act of obedience to God's will for my life and surrendering all to Him through authentic worship and prayer empowered me to focus on Him in those most intense moments, enabling me to not only endure the pain but thrive through it as well. Experiencing His Presence is converted the experience most know only as painful into a spiritual milestone.

So how do I describe and teach others how to worship in birth?

Because we are all on our own spiritual journey, we all have a unique relationship with our God; therefore how we worship may look different. Worshiping God in painful life experiences such as childbirth is not something one can teach easily, any more than teaching someone how to praise God in trials or suffering. A person who desires to worship Him does so to show her appreciation and acceptance of who God is, what He has done and is doing, and what He has promised to do. Knowing Him is the essential ingredient to worshiping Him. The only way to prepare to worship God in childbirth is to spend time getting to know Him and developing a relationship with Him that moves you to praise and worship. It's that simple.

As I was attempting to write this chapter (which I was very enthusiastic about), I found myself struggling for the right words. Since I had already shared all of my personal testimonies in the other chapters I felt it would be incomplete to not include another testimony. This struggle led me to my knees and back to the Word for guidance. Writing this book has been a labor of love for me, an act of worship to my Lord. In seeking Him and His wisdom in what to share with you, God humbled me. He revealed to me that I had forgotten some basic truths about what worship truly is. In seeking Him, He used wise brothers and sisters in the Lord, through their writings and guidance through the Scriptures, to reveal to me what was supposed to be shared here.

In order for us to worship, we need to know what worship is, right? So as I began studying what true worship was and reading about the differences between worship and praise, I realized I had a misconception of worship. Our postmodern world teaches us from the time we are young that everything in life revolves around us. The challenge I was facing in explaining worship to you came from the fact that my story involved me. It was my story, I was going to tell you what God did for **me**, share with you the attributes of God **I** met for the first time intimately, and how focusing on Him was what helped distract **me** from focusing on the pain **I** was experiencing. The problem was I was going to be teaching you about how to worship God in birth while using way too many personal pronouns.

Worship, by definition, means to adore. So to worship God means much more than to sing to Him or even to love Him. Worship is anything that includes adoring Him. Worship can include song but is not limited to it. I used to think anything we did in our lives could be an act of worship. Now that I understand true worship has nothing to do with us and everything to do with God. It takes humility and a responsive heart toward God. Worship takes intentionally leaving ourselves, our desires, needs, wants, and even our thankfulness for what He has done for us out of it. God loves it when we are thankful for what He has done for us, but thanksgiving is different from worship.

The first time I had heard of this concept of true worship was when I was introduced to Sovereign Grace's music a few years ago. If you pay attention on a Sunday morning and start counting how many times the lyrics of the songs we sing are focused on ourselves and our needs rather than who God is, you will be surprised. When we sing to the Lord are we meditating on what He does for us using the words me and I or are we worshiping Him for who He is?

God deeply desires us to bring our needs before Him, but He equally desires true worship that is not attached to selfish motives and not about us. We have been indoctrinated in our culture to constantly think about ourselves so much so that it becomes a mind game in childbirth to get our focus off the pain we are in. The only cure for self-focus is to be refocused on God alone and to concentrate on worshiping Him, to magnify Him and bring Him glory.

Kathleen Chapman wrote, "Telling God how much you love Him is not worship. It's wonderful. It's your adoration. But it involves you. True worship is adoring God alone without ever mentioning yourself . . . . Worship is one-directional. Worship is focusing on God and giving all glory to Him only, alone, singularly totally—just Him."[25]

Psalm 29:2, "Worship the Lord in the splendor of his holiness."

> "The word 'worship' translates 'God's worth.' The act of worship is focusing on Almighty God and Him alone. It's the act of assigning to God His true worth . . . . The Hebrew word *shakhah* means 'to prostrate oneself, to bow in homage, to do reverence.

This is the most common Hebrew word translated 'worship' in the Old Testament. It represents acknowledgement of who God is—His attributes, person and character. The Greek word *proskyneo* means 'to worship, to do obedience, to do reverence.' This Greek word is found fifty-nine times in the New Testament and is used exclusively for the worship of God or Christ. In both cases, worship pays deference to God alone."[26]

There are many other examples of the word worship in Scripture, but all of them refer to giving glory to God alone.

Why is it so important to understand the true meaning of the word worship with regard to childbirth? Because when preparing for your birth and for motherhood, I feel called to strongly prepare you to do more than just simply choose your favorite worship CD, thinking, "I am going to sing to the Lord in birth and my birth will be easier." Or even, "I want to experience God so I plan to worship Him in birth," while not having a true understanding of what worship is. During labor, a lot of the prayers offered up to God are requests for the Lord to provide strength, endurance, mercy, etc. The Lord wants us to cry out to Him. As our Father in heaven, He wants to bestow His blessings upon us. However, requesting His help is not worship.

Psalm 45:11 reads, "Because he is your Lord, worship Him."

The amazing reality is when you are in true worship and completely focused on Him, you are unable to focus on yourself. We talked about this concept before in the chapter "Beautiful Pain." Experiencing God through true worship helps you transcend your paradigm off the pain in birth. It doesn't come just from singing worship music, it comes from being focused on Him and adoring Him. It comes from praising His holy name and who He is. There is a place in childbirth for crying out to God for comfort, but there is also a place for true worship. He loves when we thank and praise Him for who He is and what He has done for us, but He also desires us to magnify and glorify Him through worship that is set apart from our needs and desires. When you begin as the Psalms do, with adoration, you are inviting the presence of the Lord. You are making His name known, you are revealing Him to everyone you are with in that moment as you adore Him.

To truly get your mind off yourself, you need to be in true worship of the one true God.

I greatly appreciate how delicately Kathleen Chapman shares this disclaimer in her book, which I wholeheartedly agree with, "Please do not misinterpret what I am saying. Yes we are to praise God! Yes, we are to thank Him for everything He has done for us! But we must not confuse praising God with worshiping God. There is a difference. Praise is about us—our response to what God has done for us. Worship is about God—all adoration, adulation, awe, devotion, homage, honor, reverence, and wonder for who God is and what He has done."[27]

How do you prepare to worship God in birth?

1. To be able to practice true worship, you must know God.

We can worship God by acknowledging and adoring who He is and what He has done for us, but only if we truly know Him. This is the foundational aspect for believers to worship God: they must get to know Him well by seeking the Scriptures. This goes beyond just reading a verse a day, or reading about a topic like birth. Knowing who God is and His good graces provides the foundation for a woman to worship Him in an event like childbirth where she will be challenged emotionally, physically, spiritually, mentally, and verbally. In moments like birth or any potentially life-changing event, our true nature comes out. We either praise God or we don't and some may even curse Him. You cannot be pretentious in birth—you are who you are. If you have spent time learning about who God is and practice worshiping and adoring Him regularly, then worship will flow from your heart. It is not something anyone can pretend to do at that trying time. Fear is revealed in birth, if there is fear. Faith is revealed if there is faith. Selfishness is revealed, if there is selfishness. And sacrifice is revealed from a heart that has been refined by the Father's love. It is easy for people to dress up, go to church, and smile while in church, it is an entirely different faith that it takes to worship and adore Him when the natural desire is to focus on yourself and your pain in childbirth.

Knowledge isn't worship and should not be worshiped. Having knowledge about who God is and what He has done in and of itself is not enough to lead us to worship; mere details are meaningless without understanding. Who today fully understands the Almighty? Who today has full knowledge of "I AM?" No one! But that doesn't mean we don't try to pursue God, pursue knowledge and understanding, in attempt to worship and glorify Him.

Knowing about God is not knowing God. Knowing about God helps you to better understand His deeds here on earth, but just as knowing about another person does not mean you truly know his heart, it is the same with the Lord. You can read the Bible countless hours a day, but no amount of knowledge about the Lord will ever equal having a true spiritual relationship with Him. My dear sister in the Christ, your surrender to God leads you into true worship. Knowing of Him helps you to adore Him, but if you'll just accept and know Him as your Savior that will surely lead you into worship. Our Lord does not require eloquent words, in chronological order, or themed consistency; He just wants you to acknowledge Him and surrender your life to Him.

2. Be prepared—you are going to battle me, myself, and I.

God was clearly present in my births and I was so blessed that He was. His presence was an act of His grace; it wasn't because of anything I did. So how can one invite the Lord to her childbirth? How can Christian women who deeply desire to experience God intimately in childbirth and to give Him every part of their lives prepare for this special event? By experiencing God throughout her days, worshiping and growing in her faith. Through acts of service that come from a heart that adores her God for who He is because she knows Him intimately. She speaks to Him, reads about Him, understands His Word and seeks to glorify Him by pointing to Him. Practicing these disciplines of the Christian faith is what prepares a woman to experience His presence in a new way in birth.

The central theme in our society is that birth is all about you, your body, and the baby. Because of this reality, we as Christians need to be aware of how frequently we are consumed with thoughts regarding ourselves and how we are feeling and thinking. In the stages of labor and birth, it will be an even harder challenge to keep your eyes off yourself and your pain, but acknowledging the battle is the beginning of conquering it. Prepare yourself with verses that glorify Him and are about God as well as music that helps you to cry out to Him. Talk to your husband about this concept of true worship and your desire to focus on Him. Ask him and your other birth attendants to help you keep your focus on things above and not on yourself.

While in childbirth, every Christian woman is faced with the opportunity to focus on the Lord or focus on herself. To distract your focus from yourself and the pain of labor and birth in the most intense moments, you need to exercise the discipline that you have developed to focus on worshipping God. For some, worshiping in song may be the ticket for focusing. For others it may help to meditate on Scripture or recite prayers of worship. Any way you choose is unique to your relationship with God. The key is to keep your focus off of yourself and to fully focus on God.

The Ultra-Sound of Worship

We are so blessed that the Lord created us with the ability to worship Him through song. Whether you are gifted in song or not, if you can focus on the lyrics or words expressed to worship our Creator, then you will experience being ushered into His presence.

Many of the words written and expressed through worship music, hymns, and most Christian songs point directly to His splendor. What is interesting to me is that most of the popular Christian songs talk of the most counter-cultural concepts, such as surrendering all. Yet, when we read a book or hear a speaker talk on some of the same concepts, our hearts are sinful and so quick to make excuses or justify why that isn't completely true or "doesn't pertain to me."

"You Are My Hiding Place"
By Selah
Hiding Place

"Whenever I am afraid
I will trust in You…
I am strong
In the strength of the Lord"

Why is it that songs are so quickly accepted and so quick to become popular? I believe God made us for worship. He created our bodies to feel His presence when we worship by singing, deep within our most inner being. Songs can even create physical reactions within us because we were made to worship. Have you ever been singing a song in worship, fully focused on Jesus and all of a sudden you overtaken by emotions that cause you to feel shivers? There is no doubt that true, heart-felt worship affects our whole being. Memorizing the lyrics and meditating on them is a gift from the Lord. When we recall a song it helps our focus to be uplifted and centered on Him.

> *"I will bless the Lord at all times; his praise shall continually be in my mouth. My soul makes its boast in the Lord; let the humble hear and be glad. Oh, magnify the Lord with me and let us exalt his name together! I sought the Lord, and he answered me and delivered me from all my fears. Those who look to him are radiant, and their faces shall never be ashamed ... The angel of the Lord encamps around those who fear him, and delivers them. Oh, taste and see that the Lord is good ... The eyes of the Lord are toward the righteous and his ears toward their cry. When the righteous cry for help, the Lord hears and delivers them out of their troubles."* Psalm 34:1-17

Make God Your Focal Point in Birth!

In labor and birth, one way to invite the Lord to your birth is by simply focusing on Him, praising and worshiping Him through song. Many methods teach you to choose a focal point to distract you *from* the pain in labor and delivery. My personal belief is that the only thing worthy of being focused on is the Savior and Deliverer of all pain. I am not saying it is bad to have an object like a stuffed animal or whatever you want to use, in fact, I actually have an obsession with Bounce sheets so I bring many to my birthing place and shove them into my pillowcase. I love to smell the Bounce sheets as I squeeze the pillow; they help me to relax and breathe slowly and deeply. However, the Bounce sheets are not my focal point. My focal point is Jesus Christ, which is inspired through the reading of Scripture, prayer, and worship music being played around me. In this world we live in it is uncommon for people to focus on the Lord or worship Him unless they are in a church, but He should be our focus in all circumstances. We, as the church, should be birthing our babies differently so as to shine His light on this dark world. We should be worshiping and praising Him in the good and the bad times. We should shock them with our love for children and view of them as a blessing rather than a burden. This is what sets us apart from the rest of the world; one of the ways the Lord reveals Himself to those who are lost. When you simply live out your faith in Him, as you do daily in your home, He is revealed.

Utilize Music to Create an Atmosphere of Worship and Praise!

Worship music that glorifies the Lord has the power to change an atmosphere, as well as set its tone. In our home, my children know when mommy is having a hard day or when I am frustrated, we need to put on the worship music. They know how much it impacts my attitude (and theirs); my focus is restored to the eternal rather than on the temporal. When you are in those intense moments of pain in labor, sometimes singing becomes difficult. In these moments, having music playing is especially helpful; when all you can do is simply lift your hands up in praise to the Lord. Many lyrics actually cry out to or call on the Lord, which is so applicable. I think one of the reasons why music moves me so quickly into the presence of the Lord is because I am reminded of those moments in my life, like birth, when I was empty, crying out to Him in worship and He met me there. Just hearing those songs reminds me of who He is and what He has done in my life. Remembering, appreciating, and loving Him for all He is and what He has done strengthens and restores my faith and trust in Him.

> *"Ascribe to the Lord, O heavenly beings, ascribe to the Lord glory and strength. Ascribe to the Lord glory due his name; worship the Lord in the splendor of holiness. The voice of the Lord is over the waters; the God of glory thunders, the Lord, over many waters. The voice of the Lord is powerful; the voice of the Lord is full of majesty ... The voice of the Lord breaks cedars ... The voice of the Lord flashes forth flames of fire. The voice of the Lord shakes the wilderness ... the voice of the Lord makes the deer give birth and strips the forest bare, and all in his temple all cry, 'Glory!' The Lord sits enthroned over the flood; the Lord sits enthroned as king forever. May the Lord give strength to his people! May the Lord bless his people with peace!" Psalm 29:1-11*

God Created Our Bodies to Worship and Blesses Us in Birth When We Do!

Barbara Harper, midwife and world-renowned expert in water birth, states that singing during childbirth has been the tradition in different cultures for generations.

"Hikado Suzuki, a Japanese midwife, has women practice singing during pregnancy and then encourages them to vocalize during the birth. When a woman is singing she is using her diaphragm and lateral muscles in the abdomen, which work together with the contractions. Instead of pushing the baby out, the women 'sing' out their babies. The vibration of the singing is felt by the baby, creating a harmonic resonance, which also helps relax the pelvic floor muscles and opens the pelvis. The Menahuna people in Hawaii have had a beautiful tradition of singing to the mother during her birth process. As a woman begins labor, the Kahuna, or healer, sings a beautiful

> *"I will praise you as long as I live, and your name I will lift up my hands."*
> *Psalm 63:4*

song that chronologically remembers the baby's heritage. Both midwife Suzuki and the Hawaiian people relate that labor never lasts longer than a few hours when the woman sings. As above so below—the throat is open and relaxed and so is the pelvis."[28]

Though some of these cultures are not singing to Jesus Christ, the point I am trying to make is our bodies were made to sing. We were created to worship our Creator. When we worship Him in song, He blesses us. In birth, the baby can be born faster as you focus on Him and sing with your mouth wide open, using your diaphragm.

"Let them praise His name with dancing." Psalm 149:3

Isn't it amazing that when we simply just do what we were made to do and birth babies while worshipping God through prayer, meditation of Scripture, and song He blesses us for glorifying Him by giving us strength, power, and faith in Him to endure? Having that strong faith that we can birth is essential in transition and the third stage of labor. If a woman can focus on that truth and on Jesus and the gift of her precious baby that He is about to bless her with

"Worship the Lord with gladness; come before him with joyful songs." Psalm 100:2

she will bring forth life and experience His presence in a new way. Her child's birth-day will not simply be remembered as the day her child was born, but as a milestone in her spiritual walk with the Lord because of how she experienced Him by her side all the way.

This may not be something that you experience in all stages of labor, but intuitively swaying (dancing) to the natural rhythm God designed your body to move in birth while listening to songs focusing your mind on Him is an act of praise. When we are focused on Him and our senses are alert and aware of what is going on in our body, we can surrender more easily to the way we were created to birth.

"You keep him in perfect peace whose mind is stayed on you, because he trusts in you." Isaiah 26:3

Worship through song is one way we can keep our minds steadfast on the Lord.

Resources for Worship Music

Throughout *Redeeming Childbirth* are lyrics of songs within the testimonies given.

To further equip you to have a worshipful birth, I have created a music play list with many songs that have lyrics appropriate for labor and birth to draw you into remembering the Lord, worshiping Him, crying out to Him, thanking Him, rejoicing and delighting in Him. Since most people have different preferences for music, I apologize if the music we have chosen to include isn't your preferred choice. I pray it would simply equip women with ideas and at least make their job a little easier when it comes time to prepare their own play lists for their births.

Part V

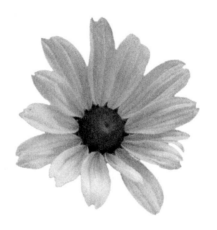

Engaging Birth and
Integrating Relationships

———❦———

Birth is a life-changing event, offering its unique impact on the lives of those involved. Obviously it is most impactful on the mother, the father, and the baby who is born, but depending on the size and closeness of the immediate and extended families and friends, this event can also affect many relationships in a deep and meaningful way.

Your birth could be a catalyst to begin a more transparent relationship with a sister-in-law, or heal a relationship with a parent. By inviting others to walk through this significant event in your life intimately with you, you will see strengthened relationships as a result. But this decision of who should be invited into such an intimate experience should be done with careful consideration and prayer. As a married couple, you should exercise sensitivity to one another's needs and hopes in choosing labor partners. The exciting thing is that God already has a plan for you and has gone before you; just seek to be open to His plan.

As women, the Lord blesses us with many different relationships in life, doesn't He? A woman can wear many hats: daughter, sister, wife, mother, granddaughter, grandmother, friend, and of course, sister in faith as part of one body in Christ Jesus our Lord.

Marriage offers many sweet blessings in life, but none really compare to the blessings of children. Your relationship with your husband will experience so much change and growth during this time of preparation during pregnancy. If you are intentional about embracing this life transition together, it could prove to potentially be one of the most impactful experiences in your marriage.

As a daughter, experiencing pregnancy and birth for the first time, you may go through a whole host of different emotions. You can create a new and special bond with your own mother, a kindred spirit of sorts, because of the acknowledgement that she went through everything you are going through to birth you. You develop a new appreciation and understanding of a mother's deep, compelling, and undying/unconditional love for her children. Daughters also have the opportunity to honor and respect their mothers (and grandmothers) by asking for wisdom and seeking their advice on childbirth and parenthood (of course filtering all through the Word of God before applying). On the other hand, many women can experience friction in their families and life transitions can be difficult because change is never easy. And for those who may not have had a mother or father around much, pregnancy can trigger a whole host of negative emotions toward their parents, including feelings of abandonment, betrayal, or even a lack of trust. The reality is, though, this life transition that comes with pregnancy actually opens the door of opportunity to experience and/or express any needed healing, forgiveness, grace, appreciation, thankfulness, and love. When one is intentional about pursuing peace and growth, the opportunity for strengthened relationships is great. It's amazing how the gift of new life and even the anticipation of it can bring a fresh perspective.

The experiences of pregnancy and birth offer all of our earthly relationships a similar opportunity for growth, though it may look different for each since relationships are so unique. As an older sister you have the opportunity to involve your younger sister in your pregnancy and birth as much as is appropriate, purposefully mentoring her and allowing her to learn and glean from your experience. As a younger sister you have the opportunity to seek wisdom and guidance from those who have gone before you. If you allow this experience to, it can bridge gaps in relationships and bring sisters and brothers together in ways that nothing else really could. Parenthood is unique in that it can bring unity and respect as well as divide and create conflict. As Christian women, though, we have the opportunity to engage our siblings purposefully and attempt to allow God to bring good out of it. Allow God to bond you together in a new way as adult siblings.

As a granddaughter, you have the opportunity to bring honor and respect to your grandparents, as mentioned above, but also to truly glean wisdom. When we as a younger generation take interest in the older, it brings such joy and delight to their lives. They feel there is a purpose. What a gift you can give your elders—worth, respect, appreciation, and honor. This is a huge opportunity for blessing.

As a mother of multiple children, every time the Lord blesses our family with another addition, the impact is significantly multiplied as well. Receiving another baby into a family is a huge life transition and impacts everyone in the household. As mothers, we have the opportunity to allow that impact be as positive as possible. For every family, how actively they pursue involving their children in the pregnancy, childbirth, and transition will vary, but there is much opportunity for immense impact on the souls, hearts, and minds of the children the Lord has already blessed us with. Teaching them, talking with them, and simply inviting them to walk through this experience along with you will have a generational impact. As parents we have the responsibility and privilege of leading our children by example. If you embrace His miracle by pursuing to surrender you birth story under the headship of Christ, inviting Him to redeem your childbirth, and if you are blessed to experience His presence in your birth, you must share that with your children.

Allowing them the opportunity to experience as much of this blessing and miracle of life as the Word guides us to, will leave a lasting impression and valuable legacy for life—teaching them by example what it looks like to invite God to be a part of every area of their lives.

As women in the church and sisters in the body of Christ, we should be proactively serving one another with regard to this common thread the Lord has blessed us to be a part of in His tapestry of life. We have a wonderful responsibility to serve one another. God has blessed us with this common thread—childbirth—which is woven through the lives of most women. The fact is, how we give birth greatly impacts who we are. Our birth stories are intimate to us and we all have them. In serving one another, we have different opportunities as the seasons in our lives change.

When we are young we have the privilege of serving young mothers by helping as a doula or supportive birth attendant or babysitter (of the other children), providing meals or helping around the home when they aren't feeling well. As we transition into the season of life when we are birthing babies, we have a new opportunity to bless the young women in our lives who are serving us. We get to purposefully teach what it looks like to be a young mom to those younger than us. If we are bold enough, we can even mentor younger women by inviting them to be birth attendants and witness our worship-led births and learn how to fully surrender to God in birth. Then, as we make the next transition in our lives to the season where we are experienced at birthing and ministering to other moms, we can teach, encourage, and equip the young mothers just beginning to have babies to embrace His miracle in birth. We can be the Titus 2 women God commands us to be.

As we embrace our new blessings and welcome them into this world through worship, praise, and prayer, we are already teaching and modeling Christ-centered intentional parenting, we are teaching and modeling for our babies intentional Christ-centered living and parenting. The journey of leaving a legacy begins during pregnancy and the eternal impact it causes is the vision to remember in the process. We need to understand that living this life intentionally surrendered under the headship of Christ means giving Him every area of our lives. There is nothing more worthy of being modeled or taught.

Every relationship the Lord blesses us with in life has the potential to impact multiple generations, especially if we cling to that vision and purposefully choose to do the hard things in life, allowing God to refine us as an example to our children and the children of others.

Let's pray together

Lord, help us to have an intentional vision with regard to our relationships. Help us allow people to be involved intimately in our lives. Bring healing in our relationships where necessary so we can fully experience all You have for us in the area of growth. Please humble our hearts to see the good in others and allow us to have teachable hearts to learn from those mentors You have put in our lives, both spiritual and biological. Thank You for our marriages. We ask, in the name of Jesus, that You would empower our husbands to be the coaches, team members, and heads of our households we need them to be. Empower them to rise up and lead our families for Your glory. Lord, help us to see the immense influence we have over our children and the next generations. Help us to raise them purposefully and lead them into a saving relationship with You. For those of us who have sisters, I pray You would give us opportunities to influence their lives. Please help us to encourage, teach, equip, and empower them as women when they come to this season in their lives. Thank You for all of the blessings You have given us in the relationships we have in our lives. Help us to be grateful for them and to treasure them, loving one another as Christ loves the church. Amen.

Birth Can Bless Your Marriage

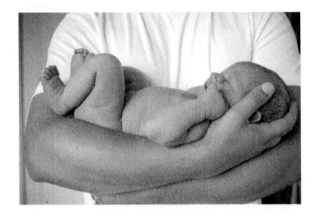

When you married your husband, God united you two with an eternal bond, "Two shall become one flesh." The making of babies is a beautifully intimate time with your husband and your Lord. This intimacy in the flesh is a gift and blessing the Lord gave you in one another. In the moment when God chose to create your child within your womb, choosing which chromosomes to take from your husband's genetics and which ones to take from yours, He "knit your child together in an intimate place." He knew your child intimately. Conception of a child is God's creation. It is a miracle, a miracle He is doing in your womb, and one that will bless and impact your life, others' lives, and eternity.

I have heard the phrase, "Making a baby is an intimate time with your husband, birthing a baby is an intimate time with your Lord." I do not disagree with this statement, but I feel compelled to share it doesn't end there.

I believe both experiences can and should be deeply intimate with both your husband and your Lord. Making a baby is a deeply intimate time with your husband and it should also be with the Lord—for He blesses your womb. Again, it takes intentionality in your relationship with your husband and God, together, to involve Him by asking His blessing upon your marriage in those intimate times. He rejoices that you are one. He made you to complement one another in this way and to Him it is beautiful to see His creation delighting in one another. But sadly, many today do not integrate God into this compartment of their lives. This time of intimacy is meant to help prepare you for the most intimate moments in the labor and birth as well.

Birth is deeply intimate between you and your Deliverer, however, you can also involve and include your husband in ways that will strengthen and build up your marriage. Laboring together and delivering your baby together can be a milestone in your marriage as well as your spiritual life. In fact, it can and should be a spiritual experience that becomes a spiritual milestone in your husband's life as well. When you choose to embrace and engage this experience together, purposefully, learning together, preparing together, and laboring together it creates a special bond that can imprint a new strength that will last forever.

God Designed You and Your Husband to Be the Ideal Team When You Work Together— Be a Team!

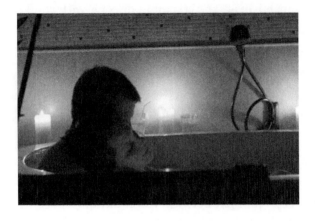

You were made to complement one another. In Genesis 2:18, the Lord God said, "It is not good that man should be alone; I will make a helper for him." Together you are made in God's image (Genesis 1:27) and given a blessing in each other. "And God said to them, 'Be fruitful and multiply and fill the earth and subdue it and have dominion over the fish of the sea and over the birds of the heavens and over every living thing that moves on the earth,'" (Genesis 1:28).

Your marriage was ordained by God and together you are better than one. Life is a journey—kind of like a long race to a finish line. There are potholes in the road, and sometimes there are injuries, obstacles, and storms. There is the temptation to give up on the race, or to just walk and be lazy, without purpose. In this race, you are given a partner, each other, to help motivate one another when you are down, to give counsel, to pray for one another, to delight in one another and God's creation, to help equip and nurture one another to be able to give your best, and to make the most of this short life we have. You are better together. Birth is one experience on your journey, and one worth preparing for together. It is like its own race.

As we covered earlier, God made your body to be able to give birth, to procreate, but God also designed your husband to be your partner in birth. Let's look at the first childbirth accounts in scripture from Genesis 4, the births of Cain and Abel.

Due to the truth that Adam and Eve were the first couple ever created, they were all alone. When Eve gave birth she had no mother or sister, no midwife, no doctor or nurse there with her to help her give birth or to take care of her after the birth. It was just her, Adam, and God. Clearly God was there with them. Eve herself praises God and gives Him the credit due for His help.

God has already given you everything you need to be able to birth your baby. He designed you, woman. He designed your husband to be your partner in birth.

> *"Adam lay with his wife and she became pregnant and gave birth to Cain. She said, 'With the help of the Lord I have brought forth man.' Later she gave birth to his brother Abel."*
>
> **Genesis 4:1**

I believe if we are looking to Scripture for our understanding of how God views birth, we must see God designed the married couple to work together as a team, like Adam and Eve, like Joseph and Mary. God has blessed us with everything we need in Him. He gave us each other, His word, and our lifeline to Him: prayer. We need to have confidence in God's design of our bodies. We need to pursue being a team with our husbands, like the examples God gave us in His Word to us. Birth is not an emergency, it is His design for procreation. It works.

As a couple, the first step toward being a team is to have confidence in His design of our bodies and the purposes of partnership within marriage with regard to childbirth. Seek Him, His Word, and seek His guidance as to where you should have your birth. Seek His wisdom as to who should be at your birth. The point is to seek Him and His wisdom, which He wants to give you.

> "Look carefully then how you walk, not as unwise but as wise, making the best of use of time, because the days are evil. Therefore do not be foolish, but understand what the will of the Lord is. And do not get drunk with wine, for that is debauchery, but be filled with the Spirit, addressing one another in psalms and hymns and spiritual songs, singing and making melody to the Lord with your heart, giving thanks always and for everything to God the Father in the name of our Lord Jesus Christ, submitting to one another out of reverence for Christ. Wives, submit to your own husbands, as to the Lord. For the husband is the head of the wife even as Christ is the head of the church, his body, and is himself its Savior. Now as the church submits to Christ, so also wives should submit to their husbands. Husbands, love your wives, as Christ loved the church and gave himself up for her, that he might sanctify her, having cleansed her by the washing of water with the word, so that he might present the church to himself in splendor, without spot or wrinkle or blemish or any such thing, that she might be holy and without blemish. In the same way husbands should love their wives as their own bodies. He who loves his wife loves himself." Ephesians 5:15-29

Your husband is assigned the privilege of loving, protecting, and providing for you. You are given the assignment to submit to your own husband and respect him. You are a team. Birth is the perfect race for a team. In your birth, you can work together to obey this scripture. Be wise, not unwise (v.15). Husbands, be wise. As you and your wife prepare for the birth of your baby, use sound judgment with regard to her health. You are her protector. Be in the Word, praying for your wife as she prepares for birth. Do not make decisions based on fear. If you experience fear of any kind, seek the Lord and His word for freedom from the bondage that can so easily entangle us in the form of fear. Do not make your wife fearful. Be strong; point her to the Lord when she experiences fear. However, part of being wise means that in the case of an emergency, and be steady. You are the part of the marriage team that calls the shots; protect your wife. Wives, don't be stubborn, obey and submit if your husband makes a decision with regard to your birthing experience (if he is seeking God and listening to Him).

"Make the best use of the time, because the days are evil," (Eph. 5:16). Make the best use of the time you have as a couple before your baby arrives in the flesh. Prepare spiritually for parenthood, prepare and work at strengthening your marriage. Deal with issues if you have them. Study the Word together. Develop habits for a lifetime like praying together. If you think it is hard to start this habit now, just wait until you have children, interrupting and waking you up. Enjoy this time, but make the most of it; be purposeful.

"Understand what the will of the Lord is," (v. 17). This is a time for you both to develop the habit of seeking Him and what His will is. "Do not get drunk" (v.18). Deal with sin. "Be filled with the Spirit . . . singing and making melody to the Lord with your heart, giving thanks " (v. 19-20). Use this time of preparation for your birth to give thanks, worship together, memorize Scripture, pray over one another, and encourage one another with words of affirmation. These

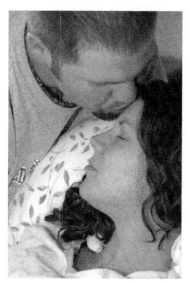

are things we are called to do anyway. It is easy to praise God in the good times, but harder when you are in pain, so no amount of practicing and meeting God in praise, worship, and thanksgiving will ever go to waste. It is beneficial so that when you are in pain in childbirth you have memorized Scripture that God has written on your heart. You cannot remember what you have not read.

Husbands, you are told to love your wives by "cleansing her in the washing of the word" (v .26). Before the birth, begin reading the Word to your wife, if you have not already. It will be uncomfortable in front of midwives and any family members who are present at the birth if you do not do it regularly at home. This is part of your role as a husband, to be the spiritual leader. Embrace it and take baby steps if you are new at it. A great thing for husbands to do to make good use time when they are preparing for the birth of their child is to do a word study through the Scriptures on fatherhood, their role as a husband, running the race, suffering, birth, pain, trials, fear, or any other topic that interests them. Search for Scriptures you can use to engage your wife when she is in birth—verses or passages that can be a comfort or encouragement to her in her pain. When the time comes, you can read them to her, or pray them over her, either laying hands on her or praying them for her internally in your head, whatever works for your wife. You need to be intuitive to her needs. What does she need? How does she want you to be involved? Ask her.

Every woman has different expectations and needs, but we are all the same in that we all want our husbands to want to be involved and we all want their support.

The Bradley Method, though not Christian, is definitely a technique that can develop strength and help prepare your marriage to approach birth as a team. It is one which your husband is actively involved and leading you as your main advocate and coach/partner.

God has tremendous blessings in store for your marriage. Obviously He is blessing you with an amazing gift—your only eternal inheritance, an heir, a sweet baby. But there is another blessing that many couples miss out on—the blessing that comes from persevering through a challenge like childbirth together. The blessing comes in the preparation, not just for your labor and delivery, but also for a lifetime of laboring in love as parents together as a team. The blessing comes during childbirth as you lean on the promises of God and He reveals Himself to you in new ways. The blessing comes in the form of growth and maturity in Him. The growth is the outcome, the effect of having relied on Him and surrendered to Him during childbirth. The growth is a blessing that strengthens and prepares you to handle the trials, storms, and seasons of this life. The growth you both experience impacts your character and your identity in Christ. It will ultimately impact generations, because your marriage will be stronger in Christ. What a fantastic blessing and opportunity for growth in marriage birth can be when you choose to proactively engage one another, growing together, seeking Christ.

It Takes Two—Preparing Your Marriage

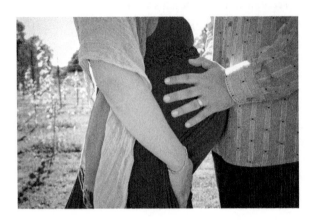

How to Prepare As a Couple for Birth

Many husbands experience a whole host of fears when they are anticipating the birth of their new baby. Whether it is his first baby or his tenth, the potential for a man to experience the stress of providing for another child and all the responsibilities and duties that go along with that, can get to him. First-time dads really don't know what to expect unless they have either been at the births of their younger brothers or sisters, taken the intiative to get educated or have been mentored by another older man with regard to childbirth. That being said, involving your husband and talking through his fears and concerns is really healthy. Remember that even though your husband is probably excited to have a baby, he is not the one pregnant and the baby is not growing inside of him. It is not on the forefront of his mind all the time. Inviting him to come to your prenatal appointments or midwifery appointments is great. Going to a childbirth education class is another great idea for preparing him for what to expect.

When it comes to choosing a childbirth education class, you need to have some standards for what to expect. Most (but not all) first-time parents are newly married and have limited funds. Because of this, many go to free childbirth classes or look up free material online. While there are certain aspects of these resources that can be helpful, I want to warn you. I have heard many testimonies claiming that secular childbirth classes offered within most hospitals are more damaging than they are helpful. I can personally attest to this as well. While there can be some value in it for the husband who knows nothing about birth, it can give him a false impression of birth and leave him with an expectation of a very limited role in the birth. This obviously can depend on the facility, so I want to give hospitals the benefit of the doubt and suggest if you cannot afford a Christian childbirth class or reading material, you should accept what is available for free. Preparing together is better than nothing, but just make sure you are filtering everything you hear and read through the Word of God and prayerfully asking the Lord to make His will known for your family.

Allow your husband to have a say in birthing choices. Ask his opinion. You might be surprised that he has an opinion. I know I was surprised when my husband became such a huge advocate for natural births. Try to learn the different labor methods/techniques and birthing options together. If he feels strongly about doing some but not others, it is healthy for you to work those things through. Read together or separately, or just give him a brief overview. Let him decide how involved he wants to be, but invite him and tell him how much it would mean to you to have him really involved.

My husband didn't catch a baby until our third child, and then he wasn't super interested in doing it again until the sixth. However, he was right there in the tub holding me and laboring with me when I gave birth to our first baby and I delivered her. Right after catching our third baby, Megan, he immediately looked up at me, leaned over and said, "We are a good team at this; we can have more." This from a man who was done after two. God had completely transformed his heart over the course of the nine months I was pregnant. I called him my "180 Man" for a long time after that third birth.

Another good way to involve your husband is when you are making your birth plan. After writing out and printing off your birth plan, verbally put your husband in charge of being your personal advocate. Whether you intend to birth your child at home, a birth at a birth center, or a hospital, it is a good idea for your husband to be mentally prepared to be both your best advocate and your baby's (in the case of an emergency). This is his role as protector. I am not trying to scare you, but just be prepared. My husband was always in charge of telling the midwife or nurse who entered the room for the first time what the plan was. It is easier on your husband if you have a plan typed or written out that they can just hand off. If you are in the hospital, it makes your husband's job so much easier if he can say, "Here is our birth plan. If you aren't comfortable with that, please get someone else to help us." Unless there are real life-threatening reasons (which there are sometimes), there should be no reason your plan cannot go the way you desire. That is assuming you have taken your plan to the Lord and are planning in His will.

Let me share something about plans. The Lord says He know the plans He has for you. He does not say you know the plans He has for you. I am a planner. The Lord has had to do a work on me in this area and the opportunity for me to have the most growth in being flexible to God's plan has been through the challenges of being pregnant and planning our births. We cannot tell without a doubt we are going to have a natural birth on any given date. But we can prepare our hearts in anticipation for the awesome works God is going to do in our births. If we don't plan to invite him, incorporate Him, worship Him, lean on Him, and glorify Him, most likely those things won't happen. If we prepare our hearts for this service of allowing God to use us as a vessel to bring forth man and we are seeking Him and desiring Him to be glorified through our births, He will be glorified. It doesn't always look the way you think it will, but God will be glorified if you dedicate it to Him. So plan and be proactive, but keep an open mind for God to do His miracles and wonders, too! Life with Jesus is an adventure. Enjoy the ride.

Birthing classes, birthing videos, and books on birth are all great ways to involve your husband in the event and to help him prepare. Just as you should use discretion in choosing your classes, you need to use discretion in the videos you watch and books you read as well. You don't want to tempt your husband into sexual sin either. Some of the videos and books available today, though they try to be tasteful about birth, are very revealing. So if you husband struggles or has ever struggled with sexual sin, I would warrant a warning toward what you watch and read. Just be wise.

Empower your husband to be your advocate, your protector, as he is designed to be. Give him guidance in how to minister to your physical needs. Communicate and try out different massages and positions before you are in labor. Read together, go to appointments together, and ask him if he would like to catch the baby or cut the umbilical cord. The point is to involve him in as much as you can. Let him be your coach and partner. You are going to be parents together so practice being a team as much as possible. It will strengthen your marriage and prepare you for a lifetime of parenting.

Praying together for you, your baby, and the birth is the ultimate way to prepare your husband for your birth. When you pray to Jesus, you just talk to Him, right? You tell Him all your fears, your hopes, your desires, all of it. Sometimes, we forget to tell our husbands these things or choose not to because we don't want to scare them, but I would encourage you to be open and honest.

Be transparent, pray together, let him see your open and bare heart. Let him hear your fears and dreams. These can be intimate times. Praying together like this also prepares him to be the prayer warrior he will need to be for you when you are in labor. Praying for you and the baby is one of his main roles as your husband in the birthing team. You need to invite him to intercede to God on your behalf and watch God answer his prayers. The times when Isaac would lay his hands on me and pray with power in the name of Jesus Christ, I experienced not only this intense closeness to my Savior and my Deliverer, but also to my husband, my earthly spiritual head. He was leading me to be strong when I was weak. When I couldn't pray for myself out loud because my contractions were too intense, he was my voice. He and I were so connected, so united as one that his prayers were my voice to God many times. The unity and closeness we experienced is incomparable to any other experience we have had in our marriage (literally shouldn't try to compare it—nothing quite like it—it falls into its own separate category—like intimacy).

My husband works hard when I am in labor. He sweats and does not stop for a nap or snack. We are a team and we stick together like one when I am in labor. He is my right hand man every time—my Mr. Steady. At the end of my birth, I have a beautiful baby, but also a glowing, truly proud husband by my side. Yes, he is proud of his new baby, but he is even more proud of me, his wife. I can see it in his eyes, in the way he looks at me.

When Isaac and I got married, like most young couples, we were head over heels for each other. We decided then the word divorce would not even be a part of our vocabulary. We also knew strong marriages didn't just happen. They were a product of work, of choices to love, forgive, and respect. We knew we would have to intentionally make time to enjoy one another when life got busy. We would have to choose to put one another above ourselves. Birth gives our men the opportunity to serve and nurture us in our pain. They have the opportunity to show us loving-kindness as they are our physical rock in birth and then our tender caregiver afterward.

One of the greatest blessings a natural birth can give a marriage is the opportunity for your husband to be very hands-on in the process. Because you are not given any numbing medications when you have a natural birth, you have full feeling everywhere in your body and can clearly move around. You are free to walk around, be in the birthing tub, on all fours, doing pelvic rocks, doing different exercises, squatting, or even dancing with your husband. When a woman has a natural birth and her body does as it was designed to do, an intuitive instinct takes over. When we don't mess with God's design, we can feel what is going on within our bodies. We are much more in tune with what is happening. In those moments when you are in intense pain, you can choose to freely move to a different position to find comfort. As mentioned before, husbands clearly have more opportunity for hands-on involvement during a natural birth. They are needed to help their wives cope with and surrender to the pain, concentrate on the baby's movements, lovingly talk to the baby, and focus on the Lord as the Rock and Deliverer. Husbands have the opportunity to lead you to worship and to spiritual reflection as your spiritual head.

Now, if a woman chooses to have an epidural, she will have to be in the hospital, confined to a bed, which greatly limits how much the husband can be involved in a hands-on kind of way. This is not opinion, it is just truth, truth that you should consider in making your decision. Also, it is medically proven that epidurals tend to slow labor down. I have heard many testimonies of women who can sleep through contractions long enough to get a nap. Often if a woman is napping, the husband is too, or he is watching TV, playing on his smart phone—anything but being directly involved in his wife's labor.

I can honestly say from personal experience, if you are in real labor (the start of which can vary among women), and you are going natural, you are not going to be napping. Some women can sleep through some of the first two stages of labor, but that is a experience that varies greatly. What we do know is God can and will provide all we need for this life if we ask Him. Sometimes it takes trying new positions out to figure out what is going to be the most comfortable position for that moment in that labor. My husband is usually very hands-on, massaging, talking to me, getting the room ready with music, my Bible, candles—whatever I want. In the pregnancies when I had back labor and posterior birth, my husband was very much hands-on. During two of my water births there was enough room for him to be in the tub with me, so he was (my first and sixth). He was rocking my pelvis, rubbing my back, pushing on my hips, massaging away Charlie-horses, rubbing my head with an iced washcloth, and feeding me ice—whatever I needed. Our marriage has been strengthened each time that we have engaged in birth and worshiped together, prayed together, leaned on and glorified Christ during birth.

When Isaac's friends ask him about the births, he always responds with praise. He aims to share certain details to build me up and to share with them how truly amazing it was. If anyone knows my husband well, they know he is a man of a few words when it comes to details. He doesn't usually take notice of the little things, but he knows I do, and he values me by noticing and serving me while I am in birth and honoring me and glorifying God during and after birth. I don't tell you this to impress you, but to impress upon you this dream, this vision, that you too can experience. I want you and your children to reap the eternal blessings that come from a thriving marriage.

Engaging your birthing experience WITH your husband can be a catalyst to a stronger marriage.

Of course it is not imperative to a good marriage, but I do believe that thriving marriages all have one thing in common: they choose to engage one another purposefully in all life circumstances, making the most of them. Birth is a major experience in life. Experience it as a team and it will make you a stronger team.

Experiencing birth as a team does not mean the husband is just there. When I say experience birth as a team, I mean labor together. Yes, the wife is the one truly physically laboring, but there is a need for the husband to engage her and be as involved as possible. When you run the race as a team, both team members have vested interests and emotions. God intends to bless marriages immensely. One way He blesses us is through the gift of children. But there is another gift that often is missed: the gift that comes in the journey of laboring together with Christ to bring forth man.

Whenever there is a trial, a circumstance in life that is hard or painful, there is the opportunity to embrace the circumstance or the pain in the moment and choose to let yourself learn, surrender to what God has in store for you with regard to growth and maturity. In your surrender, in those hard times, you will experience God's closeness. Those are the times when you can really grow. The birth of your new baby is an awesome event. It is a spiritual event because your baby was created by God. Of course, there is a sense of amazement and awe in God when you see your child being born, and that bond between husband, wife, and baby is intense and awesome. But when you have labored together, there is an added blessing. God has a gift for those couples who invite Him to journey along through their pregnancies and into their birth experiences—an eternal bond with their spouses that is almost indescribable and cannot easily be broken. The gift is the feeling of having accomplished something together that is clearly in the power of the Lord, for Him and by Him. What is more powerful than that? When you are giving birth, you know without a doubt that you are 100% where God wants you to be at that very moment. Be all there. Glorify Him and praise Him.

Dear Brother, Lead Well

A note to expectant fathers from Isaac, Angie's husband.

Hey Brother,

I came into marriage with little knowledge of anything about children, let alone pregnancy or birth. As I pictured our family, I saw two kids at some point down the road without much more thought about it.

God had a different plan than my original vision and it involved a lot of learning and surrendering to Christ on my part.

In my initial experience when Angie became pregnant, I was extremely busy building a business, and although I made it to appointments with her and tried to be supportive and there for her, I didn't get it. I didn't fully understand how important my role was. I didn't grasp that there was far more to it than listening, doctor appointments, and taking her to the hospital when her water broke.

Angie had terrible morning sickness, but being this was our first, I thought it was normal. I had a lot of sympathy for her because I had personally experienced being sea-sick for months when I went fishing in Alaska as a youth. I felt alone and depressed, so when she walked through all she did, I understood. Looking back, God was so good to have prepared me for that. I think I may have had less compassion for her if I hadn't lived through something similar.

The day she gave birth to our first child, God really woke me up. God kicked me in gear that day as I was in the tub with my wife praying with her, for her, encouraging her and comforting her as she delivered our daughter Kelsey.

Wow, what we (my wife and I) would have missed out on if we stuck to the normal process and to the pressures of the world's view of how to do this. Our marriage was forever changed for the better that day as I watched her push Kelsey out, catching her under water, and raising her to experience her first breath of air. What a special moment that I got to actively participate in. Angie truly needed me and she needed God. She put herself in a situation that forced her to fully surrender to Him. It was beautiful and my respect for her was at a new level. She could see my admiration and appreciation for her in a new way. Our marriage was strengthened as we brought our daughter into the world.

Men, I urge you as brothers: there is a real opportunity and need for us to lead our wives, especially for first-time moms. There are so many decisions to make, so many fears and emotions that can occupy their minds. Supporting your wife during this season requires a lot more than just showing up at the appointments or going through childbirth training classes. Men, we are the heads of our households and we have a unique role in our marriage. Our wives need us to be confident and steady for them in this season of pregnancy, labor, childbirth and transition more than ever. They need us to speak truth and belief in them and God's design of their bodies to do this amazing act of worship.

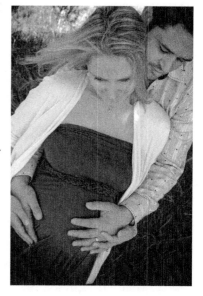

My wife was very verbal in communicating her feelings, but not all wives are. One of the things she verbalized to me was her need to know I was still attracted to her. We need to be aware as husbands that our wives go through a lot of changes while they are pregnant and their body images are very fragile, even for confident women. We need to lead their hearts and help them to know we do understand when they don't feel good or feel like being intimate, that we are still attracted to them and love them. They simply need us to cuddle them and be gentle with them. It's crucial to be there for them, not just physically there, but really present at all the right moments mentally, emotionally, and spiritually. Communicating about intimacy is an essential key to leading your wife toward having confidence in your relationship during this season in your marriage.

It is important to show deep concern for your wife, asking what her concerns are, her fears, and praying together. Reading Scripture together regularly will strengthen her and give her confidence to trust the Lord in this new experience. Whether at a hospital room, living room, or a birth center, what truly matters is that God is allowed in and is part of the process. It is our responsibility to help our wives invite the Lord into this experience. As Angie mentioned earlier, our culture has impressed upon us a set of expectations that are not always in alignment with the Bible. Once again it is our responsibility to be guiding and protecting our wives from the lies of the enemy.

It's vital we have a biblical perspective towards pregnancy. As a brother in the Lord, I would like to encourage you to simply ask yourself some questions. Test what your views are and how the culture has influenced them? Why do you believe what you do?

- How is God a part of the nine months leading up to the birth?

- What does the Bible say about birth?

- What are the pressures or fears (that either you or your wife have) that have guided the birth plan? Are you seeking your will or God's with regard to the birth plan?

More questions to discover how to be beyond the average husband

- List the ways you plan on being involved in the pregnancy and birth. Then ask yourself, honestly, if there are any things that are missing from this list that should be there.

- Where does my wife need more strength from me?

- What are my wife's fears about birth?

- How can I encourage God's involvement?

- What needs to be discussed still?

- What is my role during birth? (Husband-coached birth/team effort?)

- How does my wife like to be encouraged emotionally, physically, and spiritually?

- How am I doing at making her feel beautiful?

- What decisions is she unsure about where I need to lead?

- What family relationships are causing her to have anxiety?

- Does she feel confident about our marriage? How can I help her to feel more confident and secure?

- Is there anything I'm doing that limits absolute confidence in our relationship?

- Is there anything I am NOT doing that hurts her confidence?

It's so vital to be fully engaged in the pregnancy so she knows she's not alone. If we don't actively listen to our wive's insecurities, ideas, and questions . . . they will feel alone. She will feel insecure about your involvement, pushing her to rely on others to help instead of you.

Trust me, I know what it feels like to secretly want to be on the side-lines watching, but that's "sitting on the bench" when your needed in the game. This culturally accepted attitude is the norm today, but leads to a missed opportunity in the process of building an extra-ordinary marriage. Through showing "abnormal commitment" to your wife, leading her to trust in and pray to the Lord during the pains of childbirth you are strengthening the foundation of your marriage forever by building it on Christ.

Choosing to be involved, excited, and leading your wife helps prepare you to be more of an active father once your baby is born. Being involved in the pregnancy and birth is just as much part of the process in preparing us as it is for our wives, so engage the journey.

So, how are you going to be involved? Well, this starts the moment she tells you the good news. Your excitement, participation, and energy towards the whole process of becoming parents together will strengthen her confidence in your support. Engage her and do this as a team. Be present, ask questions, read material, and prepare together. Remember that your actions are just as important as your words. If you show her she can count on you during pregnancy, then she will have confidence she can count on your during birth (and ultimately as partners in the journey of parenthood).

Our last birth was a spiritual roller coaster when one moment I was praying and worshiping with my wife and children, the next minute I was delivering my son, and then shortly thereafter my wife was experiencing a severe post-partum hemorrhage. I am not telling you this to freak you out, but to share with you that sometimes things don't go as expected. So it is wise for us husbands to be prepared for what could potentially happen so we can make wise decisions on their behalf, if they are unable to, and so we can be a source of strength that leads them to focus on the Lord and trust His will.

Regardless of whether your wife gets ill during pregnancy, has a rough recovery after birth, or has a "text book" best-case scenario experience. This season in your marriage is one of the greatest opportunities you have to set a foundation of strength. There will be hard times in marriage and life. Marriage relationships are either growing in strength, becoming stagnate, or falling apart. We

> *"Husbands, love your wives, as Christ loved the church and gave himself up for her"*
> **Ephesians 5:25, NIV**

have to be intentional in engaging our marriages, through every life experience. How do you build a strong foundation? By following our Lord's model for true servant leadership.

When Jesus washed the disciples feet, He humbled Himself to the position of a servant. Our Lord was teaching us when He said, "I have set you an example that you should do as I have done for you. Very truly I tell you, no servant is greater than his master, nor is a messenger greater than the one who sent him. Now that you know these things, you will be blessed if you do them." John 13:15-17, NIV

All throughout this season we are given opportunities to serve our wives--to be true servant leaders. If your wife seems extra tired, let her take a nap or go to bed early and help around the house. If she isn't feeling good, ask her how you can help. And recognize that all women struggle with feeling like a failure if they can't do all that they expect of themselves in their jurisdictions in the home. Try to help them see that those things are not eternal and do your best to help lighten the load for her. Serve your wife as Jesus served the disciples. Love your wife as Jesus loves the church.

Being proactive with your wife through the birthing process is counter cultural, but it is such a powerful blessing to your marriage. It is the beginning of your journey as a parent. Once you hold your baby in your arms, your whole world is changed forever.

Lead Well,
Isaac Tolpin

The Titus 2 Call to Mentor

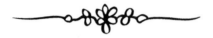

Mentoring has changed from being the responsibility and authority of the matriarch in the family, to virtual mentoring through resources online, books, and guidance from perfect strangers who have a piece of paper that puts them in a position of authority. We have been indoctrinated to value the professional's published writings over the first-hand testimonies of those closest to us. The sad response to this indoctrination is an attitude of disrespect from the younger generation for the more experienced generation. I am fully guilty of having fallen into this type of prideful attitude. In my youth, I didn't heed or even give my elders the time of day. Their words often went in one ear and out the other. It wasn't until I was pregnant with my eldest that I sought advice and wisdom from those I respected. Incidentally, I respected them not because of their knowledge, but because of the fruit of their lives, the love. We as a Christian people need to seek out the wisdom of those who we witness to have fruit, not just any fruit, but fruit that is of the Spirit.

If there were no books on what to expect when you are expecting or midwives' guides to childbirth, how would women know what to expect or how to prepare for pregnancy, labor, and birth? I am a huge advocate for midwives and doulas, and in the case of an emergency, we can praise the Lord for modern medical interventions. There is a place for doctors and surgeries without a doubt. We are very blessed God invented science and has inspired men and women to further medicine to where it is today.

Where would we be without it? However, in today's Western culture, we have truthfully lost some great aspects of tradition, respect, and purposeful mentoring with regard to family relationships. Historically, when pioneers gave birth, it was just the woman and her husband, unless she was blessed enough to have a neighbor or her mother/sisters traveling with her. Further back still, women had a strong community filled with family as well as servants to help aid in birth and recovery. They took care of one another; they helped cook food for one another and their families when there was a birth. The women within the family and community helped with births as well as deaths. These seasons in life were not avoided, but rather embraced. Wisdom and knowledge of what to expect was shared within the mother-daughter relationship, as well as family and friends. Young girls were familiar with birth, babies, and raising small children because the reality of life was not hidden from them.

In the Bible, Mary's family sent her to help her older cousin, Elizabeth, who was pregnant with John, not knowing that Mary was pregnant as well. When she arrived, Elizabeth and Mary shared a special bond because Elizabeth's baby leapt in her womb when she saw Mary. She knew Mary was with child—not just any child, but the Savior of the world. It was God's plan for Elizabeth to mentor Mary through that season of being pregnant. Mentoring is God's design for relationships. Books can be very educational. I value knowledge and enjoy reading a good book just as much (maybe more) than the next person, but nothing can compare to that real-life tangible relationship in which the secrets and mysteries of life are taught. That is why God commanded the older women in the church to be intentional in teaching the younger women in the church. He knew what would be most effective.

> "*Older women likewise are to be reverent in behavior, not slanderers or slaves to much wine. They are to teach what is good, and so train the young women to love their husbands and children, to be self-controlled, pure, working at home, kind, and submissive to their own husbands, that the word of God may not be reviled." Titus 2:3-5*

We should all aspire to be a Titus 2 woman and purposefully teach those who the Lord puts in our lives to build up. Through the years, I have had many different mentoring relationships. I am a stay-at-home mom, so I found other older stay-at-home moms who could relate and teach me on topics that would minister to my soul, heart, and mind, as well as model for me the next season in my journey. I believe strongly that even though there will always be someone older than me and it is my responsibility to seek out a mentor, I am also older than someone and it is my responsibility as an older woman in the Lord to mentor the younger women God places in my life.

How does this relate to childbirth?

I believe one of the most life-transforming events a woman ever experiences is found in the season of pregnancy, labor, and birth. Motherhood is likewise very sanctifying, but childbirth is the induction into the journey of parenthood. Yet, if you ask most women about the communication between themselves and other women on this topic of birth, especially in the Christian community, it is shocking to find that it has seemingly been avoided. Why? I think because of the division among the women in the church with regard to birthing methods and models.

Can I just share from my heart for a moment, ladies? When a woman goes to her prenatal appointments, though there is much knowledge about the process of birth, the stages, and how to prepare for them, there is no concern for a woman's spiritual preparedness. It is not even talked about. Regardless of where the baby is born, unless it is in an openly Christian center, the question as to how the new mother-to-be and her spouse would like to incorporate their faith is not even alluded too. This is why I am writing this book. It isn't the job or responsibility of the doctors or midwives to be spiritual mentors; it is the Titus 2 women who are assigned this responsibility by God.

Titus 2 women are to teach the younger women to love the Lord and seek Him in all things, including how to birth our babies in a God glorifying way. Childbirth is an intimate experience between the Lord and a woman. It is one, that when intentionally seeking Him and preparing her soul, mind, and heart for the race of birth, she can experience Him in such a way that it forever changes and empowers her spiritual walk with the Lord, equipping her for the journey in life yet to come. This is an opportunity for sanctification, and many women overlook it as such. We women in the body of Christ have an opportunity to rise up in unity and lead the women in the church. Being a Titus 2 woman doesn't offer us the opportunity to teach that which we do not live. We are commanded to teach what we are to do ourselves. Rising up and obeying God's call to be an intentional Titus 2 woman requires us to be vulnerable and real. We are to be honestly open, sharing personal testimonies and life examples as we walk through life beside our sisters in Christ.

When a young woman/girl receives the Lord, her faith journey begins. As she grows into a young woman after God's own heart, she is learning just as we did, through the study of God's Word, teachings from older women and pastors in her church, and through life experiences. The series of life events that nearly every girl dreams of follows the order of getting married and having children. Each life transition proves to be a learning experience, just as it is for all of us. When a woman gets married, she begins the journey of living and learning what it means to love her husband and learning the ropes of what it means to be a godly wife and keeper of the home. The next season in life is usually motherhood.

Being born again, getting married, childbirth, and motherhood are the four main seasons in a young woman's life. These are four of the many common threads we women have that bring us to unity. When many think of Titus 2 women's ministries within a church, they often engage teaching on faith in Christ, marriage, and motherhood, yet childbirth seems to get forgotten. Through teaching on this common experience that ninety-eight percent of women experience in life, we, the Titus 2 women, are given the opportunity to bond on an intimate level with those we mentor. It's both challenging and exciting, isn't it? To teach and encourage from a biblical perspective on pregnancy, childbirth, and the entrance into motherhood requires either knowledge of what God would want you to teach, a personal testimony of how you experienced Him in your births, or both. Are you ready?

So what should a Titus 2 woman teach on with regard to pregnancy, labor, and birth?

If we are to ask the question, "What would Jesus do?" with regard to birth, or "What would He have us teach?" then we can get to the heart of what is missing among the women in the church today.

For starters, may I suggest teaching the fundamentals:

- To spread the biblical perspective that children are a blessing from God, an eternal inheritance
- To surrender all of our lives under the headship of Christ, even childbirth
- To seek to glorify Him in all we do, including how we birth our babies
- To inspect our beliefs and abandon any lies we believe that are not from Him but rather a result of our culture's influence
- To deal with fear, and allow God to deliver us from it (fear of people, circumstances, and the unknown)
- To go to God in prayer, surrendering control of will
- To teach how to pray
- To teach how to worship (and praise Him, even when in pain)
- To invite God into every aspect of life including pregnancy, labor and birth
- To teach the truth about birth, that it is painful, but in the pain God wants to and can be your strength
- To teach that God is sovereign, holy, omnipotent, omniscient, and omnipresent

- To teach that sometimes emergencies happen, but God is still in control
- To teach faith, trust, and hope
- To teach self-control, true intent, and living on purpose
- To teach that life is NOT about us, but rather all about Jesus and to live as if we believe that
- To encourage, equip and inspire women to keep on keepin' on when life is hard
- To teach how to begin discipling their babies while they are in the womb
- To encourage women to seek God in birth, prepare their hearts, minds and souls for this experience
- To teach and encourage them to build up their marriage before this life-changing event
- To take every decision concerning the baby and the birth to the Lord in prayer
- To thank God for this great blessing, this opportunity and privilege to serve Him by raising this child for the advancement of His Kingdom
- To encourage awareness of the need and opportunities to witness to the professional health care providers during this experience
- To encourage her to prepare for motherhood
- To encourage reconciling any relationships that are unsettled
- To empower her by believing in God's ability to work through her and meet her
- To teach openness and sincerity by being vulnerable and sincere

The women mentors in the church need to be teaching a confidence in God's design of our bodies, they need to be speaking words of affirmation that are going to make a difference.

If a woman comes up to a seven-month pregnant mama and says, "Oh you look so beautiful! You are going to do great," will that truly encourage?

Does that kind of encouragement even last? Does it make an impact the pregnant woman will remember when she is in intense labor? Probably not, but it's nice to hear when your self-esteem is under attack because your clothes don't fit right. We as a church need to be speaking about the biblical promises of God's goodness, faithfulness, unconditional love, and grace, while still offering love and encouragement to these young women. Now imagine for a moment how a Titus 2 woman could encourage a younger woman whom she had developed a trusting friendship with by offering positive statements or asking her specific questions, like, "How are you doing preparing spiritually for birth? Have you thought about your birth plan? Tell me about it . . . . Have you considered how you might incorporate your faith in birth? You know, Jesus loves you so much that you are going to do great. Have you ever thought about how God wants to be your strength when you are weak? God made your body to do this good work, have faith in Him. If you would like to pray for your birth together or study childbirth together, I sure would love to do it with you!" Wow, if intentional mentoring was happening in churches across America (and the world), and truth was being taught, and conviction encouraged just imagine what would happen. Imagine the generational impact this would have on the legacy of faith from these young mothers who are raising our next leaders!

These things need to be modeled and taught intentionally to the next generation because they have been overlooked for too long. God chose older women as teachers knowing they would have been humbled through the sanctifying experiences of marriage, pregnancy, labor, birth, and motherhood. The Lord has called us to model living a life of submission to God through personal testimony, teaching, prayer, and acts of service. When a mom is on bed rest and you offer to come watch her kids, bring her a meal, or clean her toilets, your actions become teachable moments.

Once you have given birth, you have something to teach younger mothers-to-be who have not. But take this charge seriously. Your responsibility is to build up your younger sister, not scare her. You are to teach what is good and will encourage her to live in submission to God's will for her life. Remember her birth story is going to be unique and that is God's beauty at work; it is not supposed to look just like yours.

What we as Titus 2 women should strive to teach them about birth is to experience Jesus, to lean on Him, to worship Him, pray to Him, and to be humble and open to whatever He has in store. We should teach the younger women God wants to meet them there and show Himself to them in a new and powerful way. We should teach about all the ways God might want to redeem their births. In surrendering her birth experience to His will, God may really want to reconcile family relationships, strengthen her marriage, witness to a nurse or midwife, or simply minister to her and reveal Himself to her in a more personal way. Showing her how to pray and seek Him through His word will help guide her toward God's will for her life for her birth experience.

We should all be striving to be Titus 2 women and looking for opportunities in our relationships to build one another up toward good works and faith in Jesus Christ.

Questions a Titus 2 Woman should ask

1) Who has God put in my life that I should be more intentional with?

2) Who can I ask to mentor and help me keep growing in the Lord? Looking around at the women in my life, who has fruit I respect?

3) Am I mentoring my own children well in the Lord? In order to be teaching others, we should reflect on our own homes first. We cannot be those who believe "If you can't do it, teach it." A good spiritual thermometer is our children. Go to them and ask them for honest feedback. (This one is convicting.)

Being an Intentional Sister

As an older sister, I used to think my job was to be the role model to my younger siblings. I'm sure you know what I mean—if you have children you've probably said it yourself, "You are setting an example for your brothers and sisters," when they do good or bad things. Growing up though, I don't believe I was a very good role model. I was moving out and up north to a university when my sister was just shy of seven years old. She admits she barely remembers what it was like when I lived at home. In high school I was self-absorbed with sports, work, friends, and extra-curricular activities. Even when I lived at home, I was never really there much.

Growing in my relationship with the Lord made me realize that I was to do more than just be a role model. I was to be purposeful in my relationships with them. Unfortunately, I was geographically far away and on a budget due to college costs. Then, when I did come home for summers, I had to work to pay for college and missions trips and still was too busy. Sadly, I had missed the opportunity to develop real friendships with my siblings.

Years later, I was pregnant with my second baby, and I wanted to share this experience with my sister who was ten years younger. I felt it would be good for her to witness how babies were born. I thought every young lady should know. But I also deeply wanted to share this special experience with her and for her to get to know me more intimately. I was purposefully trying to mentor her and share this sacred event in my life with her.

I was overdue by one week and went in to the hospital to be induced. I was not aware of the implications of being induced, like how it can make labor much harder and faster. Regardless, I had been dilated to four centimeters for nearly three weeks and was having really intense back pains that were preventing me from sleeping for two of those weeks. Needless to say, when the midwife suggested stimulating labor by breaking my water, I was all for that. My husband had been traveling a lot with work and I was really worried he wouldn't be in town when I went into labor. Considering all the circumstances, getting induced seemed like the wisest option. I wanted to labor in the water and have a natural birth again, but I was concerned that if I lost anymore sleep I wouldn't have enough energy to birth this baby on my own.

So Tuesday morning I went in to be induced. They fed me a big lunch, broke my water and we waited for about two hours and nothing happened. I realized in that moment how risky inducement was—even at four centimeters dilated—when the midwife came back in and said, "You have twenty-four hours to have your baby and then we will need to talk about a caesarean." Talk about pressure! Shortly after breaking my water, my mom and thirteen-year-old sister showed up at the hospital. When they realized I wasn't progressing, they went down to the cafe to grab a bite. While they were gone, I felt contractions coming on. So I jumped in the birthing tub. I wanted dibs on that bad boy and there was only one to share in the whole hospital.

Isaac put worship music on and we prayed while we waited for the contractions to pick up. Within an hour and a half I was in transition and burning up hot. I chose to get out of the tub because it was too hot, so I had to do the rest of my laboring in my room. My mom and husband massaged my back as I was having terrible back labor. Being out of the water made the pains in my back worse, but I was already out and couldn't imagine climbing back into that thing and waiting for it to fill back up.

The waiting was short because my contractions were the most intense of all my births. I remember how hard it was to say a simple word between those contractions! I would randomly spit out one word at a time like, "pray," "ice," "Thank . . . you . . . Jesus," and "baby." Then suddenly, just two hours after my more gentle contractions began, I was pushing. Austin came so fast the midwife had no time to put her gloves on. Only having had enough time to get one leg in a stirrup, my mom held my other leg. Every time I pushed my leg I would also push her away on a wheeling chair, leaving us laughing. I remember laughing so hard I was crying, but maybe I was crying because of the pain and laughing because of the look on my mom's face.

After my first push, I remember my mom asking my sister if she was ok. I remember thinking to myself, "Hello, I am the one giving birth here." I will never forget the look on my sister's face just as I was about to push for the second and last time. She had a glazed over look on her face and I was afraid I had scared her. I glanced back at my husband and just looking at him refocused my attention back on the task at hand. I was about to hold my sweet baby in my arms. Immediately after Austin was born and he lay in my arms gazing up at me and my sister right by one of my shoulders, my mom asked her again if she was ok and she said with a huge smile, "Yes, I am fine. That was amazing." She went on to express to me how it was the most incredible event she had ever seen.

I was so relieved to hear her express such deep appreciation for being there; it made it all worth it. I was worried I had scared her out of ever having children, but she actually began thinking about wanting to be a midwife afterwards. Though that never became her career, it spoke volumes to me about how much of an impression it made on her.

In life, we have few opportunities to share very special and intimate moments with our siblings. I am so glad I have had the opportunity to share three different births with my sisters.

Birth has truly brought the women in our family together, closer than before. I wouldn't have it any other way. I know they have seen my heart, my love for my children, my love for the Lord, my love for my husband, and my love for the gift of life. I know they know the real me. I have not withheld anything from them.

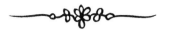

A Sisters Bond
Kathy & Lindsay's Story

I am so blessed to share this beautiful testimony of natural family mentoring between two sisters-in-law.

"When Kathy got pregnant, I was already about four months pregnant and was so excited for her and my brother-in-law. Kathy was not from a family familiar with natural or home birth, and she was pretty scared. Months went by and we had the opportunity to share our birth testimonies and resources and I offered support in any way she needed. I was so honored when she asked me to be one of her birth coaches/doulas, even though she had planned on having a hospital birth and I had never had one and didn't really know what to expect. Then came time for me to give birth. I labored in the tub outside in the back yard while the little ones played on their bikes and with their toys. It was a really difficult labor, probably my hardest, and I was really nervous I would scare Kathy because she was due in just a few months and had never seen a live birth before, but it bonded us in such a sweet way. There were so many women from both sides of our family there, it was like a community gathering. The camaraderie that was bred between us all was so strengthening for our whole family.

A few months later, Kathy's turn came, and we headed off to the hospital. She did a fantastic job. I was so impressed with how everything went at the hospital. I think I had a wrong impression of what to expect and I was pleasantly surprised. You can have a very special natural birth in a hospital." Lindsay

"I was born and raised in Michigan where traditionally babies are born in the hospital, not at home. In fact, when my mother-in-law and sister-in-law started sharing with me about natural birth I was really nervous, but the more information they gave me the more confident I became. It really helped that my husband had been to four of his mom's births. He said it took an unnecessary mystery and anxiety out of childbirth. Whenever I would get nervous he would say, "Don't worry about that." His confidence in me and in my body to birth our son made me calm and gave me peace.

I was so thankful when Lindsay invited me to be at her home birth. I had never been to a birth before and it wasn't scary at all. Being there gave me a sense of confidence that my body was designed to do this, just as she did what she was designed to do. When I first found out I was pregnant, I thought I would probably have an epidural in the hospital for sure! I thought, "Why would you ever have your baby at home?" Everyone I knew had epidurals and hospital births; it was just what everybody did. I didn't want to have to go through pain if I didn't have to. I remember when I told my mom I was seeing a midwife, she was supportive but confused. Why I wasn't seeing a doctor? After all, that was the way everyone did it back home. I was really nervous to have a natural birth. By the time the baby was due I had talked to a lot of friends who had natural births, I had been to birthing classes with Nathan, and I had witnessed Lindsay give birth. Our families were really supportive. I was so blessed.

The best advice I received was to make the decision on where to have your baby in prayer and where you feel you have the most faith, so that you are not extra nervous or stressed out. For us, I felt most comfortable in the hospital. We prayed a lot about this birth and the Lord was there. God placed awesome nurses in our room. The second best advice we had was to make a birth plan.

During the actual birth, I labored for hours. Lindsay and Nate were with me. They were so great at working with me. Lindsay really helped with getting me to try different positions and move around. I was exhausted and lethargic so they gave me an IV for fluids. Then came time to push. After pushing for two hours, the doctor was considering using the vacuum and then I pushed him right out. I was so relieved it was over, but then they whisked him away because he had meconium in his throat. I didn't get everything I wanted on my birth plan, but the things compromised were pretty minor in the grand scheme of things. In the future, I might be open to home birth, now that I have done it naturally once. The idea is warming up to me.

Overall, I am so thankful and blessed to have such an amazing family and support system. Even though many of them are huge natural birth/home birth advocates, their love for me was apparent. I never felt judged by any of them for having a hospital birth. They were so good about mentoring me and I am so glad they did. My birth experience was totally different than it would have been I am sure." -Kathy

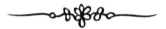

These women are family because their husbands are brothers, but they are also sisters because of their bond in Christ Jesus and their bond as mothers who have shared an intimate and cherished experience in life together. It brings tears of joy to my eyes to dream of my daughters and daughters-in-love having those close relationships. Because of their testimony of intentionality, authenticity, and sharpening one another as iron sharpens iron, I dream bigger for my daughters and their future relationships. What a beautiful picture of family, of sisters, of natural mentoring. I am so blessed to have interviewed these sweet young mothers. Thank you ladies for sharing your story.

Mentoring Mothers

Our mothers are God's gift to us, just as you were hand picked by the Lord to be your daughter's mentor.

God has chosen natural mentors we should not overlook. Just as He chose you to be your baby's mentor, He also chose your mother to be your mentor.

Nothing compares to having your mother as a birth mentor and support when you give birth. They are equal blessings but obviously entirely different experiences. No one can be more in tune with your needs than your mother. Moms simply know us better than almost anyone. And because they can sense our needs so intimately, they are the best prayer warriors when we are in birth, pain, or in any other circumstance in life. No one has the ability to build you up more quickly than a mother. When a daughter hears words of affirmation from her mother, it is extremely powerful. In general, there is something powerful in hearing words of affirmation and encouragement from fellow women who have run the race of childbirth.

Mothers are God's gifts to daughters in that they are His chosen mentors. As young women, we need to understand that just as God chose us to be our daughters' mothers, so He chose your mother to be yours. Just as in parenting we learn much about ourselves and our sin, and are refined by the life experience of parenthood, so are our mothers. In any mentoring relationship, the learning and teaching go both ways. I learn so much from my children. Every day they show me how sinful I am, but it is a reality I wouldn't change for the world. They make me a better person and keep me humble. As mentioned earlier in the chapter on prayer, having your mother there at your birth to pray for you enables her to walk through a very necessary life transition.

The life transition from mother to grandmother is one I greatly anticipate one day, but there is not much teaching on how to go through this transition gracefully. Media portrays pregnancy, birth, parenthood, and the relationship between grandmothers and their daughters completely brash. Certainly you have heard the jokes about good Ol' Gram and how she can't let her daughter be the mom, always telling her what to do and butting her head into places she shouldn't. Why is this? I believe it is because respect is missing from today's families. Respect goes both ways. Many have said to get respect one must earn it. Let's see what God's word says:

> "Do not withhold good from those who deserve it, when it is in your power to act." Prov. 3:27, NIV

> "Pay to all what is owed to them: taxes to whom taxes are owed, revenue to whom revenue is owed, respect to whom respect is owed, honor to whom honor is owed."
> Romans 13:7

> "Show proper respect to everyone: Love the brotherhood of believers, fear God, honor the king." 1 Peter 2:17, NIV

> "Honor your father and your mother, so that you may live long in the land the LORD your God is giving you."
> Exodus 20:12, NIV

I believe when you as a daughter respect your mother and allow her to be a part of your birth process, something transforms in her heart and it will help her to give you respect as a mother. It is part of the life transition God designed her to walk through—the realization that you are also a mother now. All mothers struggle with allowing their babies to grow up in one regard or another. Some do not need to be at their daughter's childbirth to realize this, but for others it could prove to be very powerful. When a mother is allowed to witness her daughter giving birth, I believe it not only strengthens their relationship, but brings the new grandmother to a conscious realization that her daughter has grown up. God designed mothers to nurture. That deep and God-instituted nature does not disappear the day her daughter is married. I believe this innate desire to care for your children will never die.

"My mom has been at all of my births, to support us in any way possible, whether she was playing with the little ones or praying over me. During my first birth, just as I was near ten centimeters dilated, we received the unexpected news that our baby was breach. The Lord knew. Once the midwife realized the fullness of the situation the room went quiet. I felt perfect peace in her abilities. She seemed very much in control and confident—another one of the Lord's mercies. I knew if we had been in the hospital we would have surely had a C-section. Thank you Jesus! In one area of the room, I noticed my mother, praying in tongues. She knew the only way she could help was by praying for me, so that was what she did." -Lindsay Edmonds, PassionateHomemaking.com

Family dynamics are not the same everywhere

Having your mother at your birth is not for everyone or every circumstance. I understand many women today are not blessed with good relationships with their mothers; in fact many come from very dysfunctional relationships and some have even been deserted by their mothers. First of all, let me just say my family is not perfect. If you asked my mom she would openly admit our relationship hasn't always been the ideal mother-daughter relationship. However, we try. Sometimes we hurt each other, sinning against each other, but we also apologize and forgive one another. I try to respect my mom by including her in intimate moments like birth, and when I do, the Lord blesses our relationship immensely.

Whether or not you invite your mother to be a part of your birth is something you really should pray about and decide with your husband. Just as mothers have the power to encourage and build up in such an intimate way, they equally have the power to discourage and tear down. There are many things to take into consideration when deciding on your birth attendants, including: your relationship with your mother, your husband's relationship with your mother, how does she handle seeing you in pain, is she controlling, is she going to be encouraging? These are all questions one should ask, but in this process of deciding, don't forget to take it to the Lord in prayer. He may have a different plan than you do and His plan is always the best. In fact, you may not understand it now, but God may have some relational healing in store for your relationship if you allow Him to do what He wants.

I had the blessing of being able to have my mother at four of my births and my mother-in-law at two of my births. The encouragement they were able to give through having pure confidence in me, in my body's ability, which was created by God to give birth, was most empowering. There were moments in my first birth when I would look into my mother's eyes and instead of her eyes showing fear, there was strength and power. I felt a stronger bond with her that day. She knew what I was going through and had survived it herself. I knew I would survive as well. No matter how old we get, there are those moments when having your mother present just makes the experience. Birth is one of those times.

It was not an easy decision for me to invite my mother-in-law to my birth and to this day, I do not know many who are willing do this. What was my motivation? My motivation came from the Lord. After having bonded with my own mother and sister in my first three births in such a special and spiritual way, I desired to have that same growth in my relationships with my mother-in-law and sister-in-law as well. My mother-in-law, Sarah, is a very sweet woman who loves her children deeply. I felt the Lord prompting me to share this intimate experience with her as well as my sister-in-law, to allow them to know me more intimately, as well as experience the Lord together in birth.

I wanted them to know the real me, not have this picture of who I am when things seem good, easy, and joyful. What more authentic way for someone to witness your convictions and beliefs in action or get to know you more intimately than in a life transition like childbirth? When in the midst of pain in childbirth, you cannot fake who you are. Out of our hearts comes the truth about our faith and I had experienced God most intimately in my births so I wanted to invite them to experience what I had first hand with me. When you can intentionally invite those you love most to be involved in such a spiritual experience and grow with you—why wouldn't you? So I invited them to experience His presence there with me. Since I had already opened myself up intimately with my mother and sister, I wanted to be fully transparent with both sides of our family.

I wanted them to know the real me, the one obsessed with worshiping God. I wanted them to see the side of me that cries out to Him with tears of joy while enduring the pain of childbirth; the me who struggles with fear and has to continually surrender it to the Lord; and the me, who just like every woman, gets to the end of her rope sometimes and needs another sister to remind her of the end prize. I truly believe that because I have opened myself up in a very intimate way to all the women in my family they know me and have witnessed our Lord in action.

I recognize how blessed I am to have mothers who desired to be involved in my births. Unfortunately, there are many women who do not have that blessing. This is another example of an opportunity for us as the church to minister to one another and to be deeply involved in one another's lives. When a friend goes into labor, offer to watch her children, stay with her until her husband gets home from work, or even be available as a birth attendant. Whatever the case, we are the family of God and should act as a family. This is an opportunity for surrogate spiritual mothers to step up and fill a void, ministering to the younger sisters in the Lord.

The point I want to drive home is that we women need each other. God has blessed us with family and with the family of God, so let's collaborate in this spiritually significant life transition into parenthood.

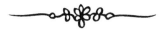

Dearest Grandmothers to be

Nearly twelve years ago I began the journey of being a grandmother. Was I prepared? No. Was I anxious? Excited? Nervous? Yes.

As I recall being present with my daughter, Angie, for the birth of her first child, I remember the James passage above. It says, "Every good gift and every perfect gift is from above and comes down from the father of lights . . ."

"Every good gift and every perfect gift is from above, and comes down from the Father of lights, with whom there is no variation or shadow of turning," (James 1:17, NKJV).

I look back on my experience of being a mom,"walking through a messed up knee from volleyball with my daughter Angie, a broken leg from snowboarding with my son Tim, and a few broken bones from roller-skating with my daughter Katie . . . . I held the kids in my arms and in my heart with prayer as I tried to relieve their pains and encourage their hearts about life on the other side of these momentary afflictions. Most mothers have had these moments of nursing a child through pains, but being present at the birth of a child is a unique experience that is unmatched by any other. It is "Every good gift from above coming down from the father."

It was my first experience at a birth—my daughter's first—and I was to be present as a second support person. I am not sure if I supported her or if we supported each other. I remembered my own birth experiences, and had a sense of what was coming, but watching a daughter labor is joy and agony in each breath and contraction. I remember wishing I could remove the pain of childbirth from my daughter (it is so hard to see our children in pain), but also thanking God that I could not do that. I thanked God for each contraction, for each time the midwife said you are dilated to four or five and then finally ten, knowing each pain was bringing my daughter closer to a joy beyond all measure. Being present allowed me to comfort her and encourage her heart, helping her know she would make it through this experience and be led into a more joyful experience—the blessing of motherhood.

During my time with my daughter, I was able massage her back, be an ice chip runner, pray for her when she was weary, and pray for God to bring the baby into the world safely and quickly. God has been faithful in hearing my prayers for my daughters as they labor and anticipate the good gift from above which they are receiving. The moment of birth is such a time of joy for all those present. I found myself tearful at the realization that not only was I greeting a new grandchild, but my own daughter was also moving into a new era of responsibility that would change her life forever. My life was changed forever too.

Only two weeks ago, I was invited to share for a part of my daughter-in-law's first labor and birth experience. It was also a special time for me to help her know when she felt weary that it would end soon and that she was brave and strong and able to do the task before her. It was also a time of prayer—asking God to bring the baby quickly -- because I could not take away the pain from this young woman who is so dear to me. Once again I found myself massaging her and grabbing a bucket for her when necessary, getting a glass of water, helping her find different positions that might give her a tiny respite from the pains which were so intense. I hope my experiences of just being, loving, caring, and sharing the moments of labor and delivery will encourage you to consider being there if and when your daughter or daughter-in-law asks for you to do that.

I know it could have been a stressful time if I went in with answers for every problem or advice on every contraction. I knew God's plan for me was only to give encouragement in whatever direction the parents found they needed to go as the labor progressed. If there is any advice I can stress, it is this—go in with an open heart and a mouth that only speaks support for the mother and father who are walking through the birth experience. It is not a time to be in charge of the situation. It is a time to submit to God and ask Him to use you in a positive way to help your daughter through the job of labor and delivery and give thanks with her when you finally get to hold the precious baby which you have all waited expectantly for.

When my daughter-in-law invited me in, I entered and she said to me, "This is not what I expected, but I don't know what I expected." I reassured her there is no way for a woman to explain what to expect in labor and delivery, the experience is unique every time. We cannot always prepare our children for what they are going through but we can support them and encourage them when the going gets tough. A word of caution here as well, I made the mistake of sharing how easy a couple of my births were (two and three—not the first!). That probably was not a fair thing to share on the first birth experience for my daughter-in-law. The first birth is often the hardest and longest trial. Our job is to help them see the light at the end of the tunnel and rejoice with them when they arrive!

The experience of childbirth is special every time because God is blessing us with a gift from above. I have had the opportunity to be present for the arrival of five of my seven grandchildren and I would not trade that experience for anything in the world. It is a time of loving your daughter, embracing a grandchild, and growing together through an experience that will never happen again exactly the same. Each time I have watched a birth experience, it has been different. Each time I have found myself thanking God for my daughters, their courage, and their love for me—to include me in watching God's creation take place in our midst.

I have found no greater joy than being present for the births of my grandchildren and holding them in my arms for the very first time. What a gift to see the wonder of God's creation. May you be encouraged to accept the opportunity to walk through this experience with your daughter one day and may God strengthen your relationships as He has ours because of it.

Blessings,
Vicki Knutsen

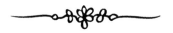

Both of my mothers have been great examples of quiet, gentle, supportive, servant leadership at my births. In my first birth, my mom was there, available to help and encourage in any way she could, but she also gave my husband and me respect by giving us space to labor together. I knew she was there if I needed her, but she really amazed me at how self-controlled she was as a first time grandmother. When my mother-in-love came as a birth attendant, she was likewise very behind the scenes, helping when she could, patiently. But when I needed her, as an older woman to speak bold truth into my soul with confidence, she was there ready to fulfill that need. There was a point when I was fearful I couldn't do it. I felt for sure the baby was stuck and I was exhausted. Sarah grabbed my hands, looked at me in the eyes and firmly said, "You can do this." That was exactly what I needed to hear at that very moment. That moment bonded us as I pushed him out minutes later. Their strong but graceful support and love were all I needed, and exactly what they provided.

I have to say, looking over the years at my mothers, they have never been ones to involve themselves in our parenting decisions unless we ask. I hope I can be just as supportive and respectful of my children and their spouses when I am a grandmother.

Purposefully Mentoring Your Daughters

All throughout Scripture, God's chosen people, the Hebrews, were sanctified through punishment, nations overtaking them, etc. Then God would have mercy on them and deliver them, commanding them not to forget what He had done for them. He had commanded them to teach the next generations the history of what He had done, lest they forget. And yet, in their humanity and forgetfulness, they would forget, and the next generation wouldn't remember, and they would grow further from God and the truth and the way. We as a Christian body need to learn from their example and get back to allowing God to sanctify us, not just for our own righteousness and refinement, but for the future generations, that we might stand up and bless the Lord by telling of the good works He has done in our lives. We need to share His story with our children so they might believe and serve His Kingdom.

It is a rare opportunity when we get to allow our children to be the spectators in our sanctification. Embracing this opportunity for growth and being challenged to practice self-control while our children are watching will have a generational impact. I guarantee the children will not forget too quickly what they witnessed.

In our pain, He wants us to draw near to Him. He wants us to tell the story of His deliverance in our lives. Jesus desires for us to experience Him intimately. His protection and presence in birth is one way we can. The Lord wants mothers to share their stories with their daughters, and in so doing, leave a legacy of faith. God commands Titus 2 women to stand up and empower the younger generations toward good works through teaching and walking through life's seasons together. We are to share in this special life journey, older women encouraging the younger women to pursue God and holiness and submitting to the Father's will in every area of life including childbirth.

What better place to begin than with one's own daughters?

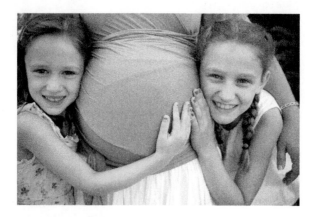

Let's not be mothers who preach, "Do as I say, not as I do."

Instead, let's let our actions speak loudly for themselves as we teach our daughters how to birth gracefully, leaning on the Lord.

Communicate with your mother/or daughters about your expectations

Talking with your mother or mother-in-love about your expectations BEFORE your birth is very important!

Here are a few questions for you to think about with regard to what you should talk through:

1) When do you want her to meet you at the hospital, birth center, or at your home?

2) Who are your primary and secondary labor coaches? What are their roles?

3) Share your birth plans with her by giving her a copy of your plan and maybe even this book so she knows what you are expecting and hoping for. Ask her if she has any questions.

4) Explain to her what you envision her role to be. Take time now to write thoughts down. Do you want her to be in the background running for ice chips, praying in the corner, helping with the other children, or on her hands and knees helping massage your back and singing worship music with you? Dream . . . what do you envision?

5) Ask her what she envisions. Sometime during your pregnancy, ask her about her birth story. This may potentially be a very sensitive subject depending on her experience or comfortability with being vulnerable on such an intimate level. Remember to have grace with her as well as other family mentors in your life. If you tend to fear birth and you know she has not healed from or dealt with a traumatic experience she had, it may or may not be wise to approach that until after you have given birth.

6) Plan to communicate about your birth again before the due date. Communication is key to having realistic expectations.

Leaving a Legacy

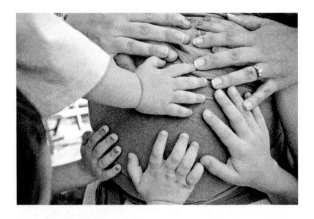

Becoming parents is a beautiful gift from God. From the moment of conception there is a physical, spiritual, chemical, and emotional connection between a mother and her child. God designed our bodies so that we would enjoy a growing bond with our babies all through pregnancy. When you are pregnant, you have the opportunity to teach your baby about the Lord as you worship, as you read the Word of God aloud, as you pray, and as you converse with others. Your baby can hear. Your baby is listening to how you treat your other children, whether you are in tender cuddling moments or in moments of correction, your baby is listening and learning about you, his/her other family members, and about his Father in heaven. He is learning what kind of mother you are to your other children. Humbling thought, isn't it?

After birth, we hold our babies for the first time, cuddling them to our bosoms, skin to skin, nourishing them naturally and tenderly. Many books and studies validate that the first few hours with your baby are critical in developing trust and a healthy bond with your baby. I would like to suggest that as purposeful parents we take every hour we have with our children as opportunities to develop a healthy bond. Pregnancy and childbirth are not the pinnacle experiences in your relationships with your children. They are the beginning of many experiences. You want to pursue giving your best to your child not just in pregnancy and childbirth, but every day you are so blessed to have the gift of their presence in your life. Pregnancy and childbirth are preparing you for a lifetime of laboring in love for your children.

As your children grow, and God adds more children to your family why not take the opportunity to involve them—to be blessed and mentored during the birth of their siblings and increase their understanding and appreciation of God and His design. Instead of keeping your pregnancy and childbirth exclusive to just you and your husband, what if God would like you to incorporate family more and use this time as a teaching tool in your children's lives. God wants us all to purposefully teach our children not to fear Him but to embrace His will. By not involving your children you are teaching them that pregnancy and childbirth are so personal and private it is not for them to be a part of. You are potentially (not necessarily, but potentially) teaching them to fear it or to avoid talking about it. As parents, we are either teaching them to be open and able to freely talk about things or to bottle it up/feel uncomfortable talking about it. Birth is intimate, but we need to bridge this gap and start purposefully teaching that birth is intimate in a way that brings glory to God. Your children can grow not only in their relationship to you, but also in their understanding of how our Creator has designed their bodies intricately and perfectly to make babies and give birth.

Don't mistake me—I am not suggesting the only way to engage your children and teach them about this miraculous event is by having them there. Not at all! I have not had all of my children at my births. I personally believe it is something that needs to be prayerfully considered, with careful concern for each child on an individual basis as well as considering what you may feel God leading you towards for the vision of your birth. The point I would like to make though is that if we can openly converse with our children, at their individual levels of understanding and try to allow them to be as involved as possible . . . it will not only teach them about pregnancy and birth, but it will eliminate many potential fears they might have and help them to view birth and intimate topics like it in a different light allowing them to have better communication throughout their childhood.

The more we utilize this opportunity to engage in teaching them about life, the more vivid a memory it will be for each child. My hope would be that you would at least consider the benefits to involving your children more, pray about it with your husband, and make a decision together. But know this—whatever you choose to do or not to do will leave a lasting memory with your child. It will leave a legacy, intentionally or unintentionally.

In Deuteronomy 6-10 it says to teach God's commands to your children while you walk, sit, lie down, etc. He also says to remember to tell the stories (His story) of what He has done in the lives of their fathers. The Bible does not specifically say to teach them as you give birth, but obviously this is how young women learned how to give birth at such a young age back in the biblical days. Back then, families of women were much more intentional in passing down teachings from one generation to another because they often lived together. We miss out today because of our western culture's desire for independence and individualism. So we mothers and fathers need to fight a cultural battle to preserve what God intended to be the natural means of teaching from one generation to the next. We need to pursue allowing our children to be with us as often as possible. Faith is not taught, it is caught. Teach them faith as they live through some of the trials, challenges, and growing experiences in your life. Don't shelter them from it all. I am not just referring to birth here, obviously. This goes for any experiences we have in life. Are we humble or vulnerable enough to share our failures and hardships with our children in a way in which they'll glean depth of faith and trust in our Savior? Childbirth is just one experience of many in our lives where we have the opportunity to be purposeful in mentoring our children. Allow God to work in their young hearts so they can stand on the shoulders of their ancestors, elders, mentors, and parents.

Today we label children and set low expectations for what they can understand, comprehend, and do. We need to take those expectations to the foot of the cross and ask God to reform our philosophies of parenting and transform our minds to be more like His. We need to choose to be parents who aren't scared to learn things with our kids. We need to be humble and lead our children in humility. There is nothing more humbling than giving birth with your children right there next to you. Be a humble leader, allowing your life lessons to be their classroom as well. There is nothing like firsthand experience. I believe if more parents were transparent with their children and openly communicative, inviting the child to be involved in the birthing process to some degree, there would be many more children with a deep connection to God. There could be a revival among the young people in Christian homes today. I know from my personal experiences with my children who have been at my births that God has blessed those relationships with a rare respect.

When anyone witnesses a child being born into the world, they can't help but be in awe. But as a child, watching a sibling being born adds a depth of respect between that child and her mother. I remember how proud Kelsey was of me the first time she saw me give birth. No other experience in life could quite compare to that, just as no experience in life can quite compare to the sibling bond that is tied when one sibling watches another being born.

I remember the look on Kelsey's face when she saw her brother Luke being born. There are no real words to explain the sweet relational bond between the two of them. As she held him for the first time, she had this cute smirk on her face, like she wanted to shout, "WOW I LOVE

YOU SOOOOOO MUCH BABY," but instead she contained herself to holding him quietly, gently, and tenderly while she sat in awe.

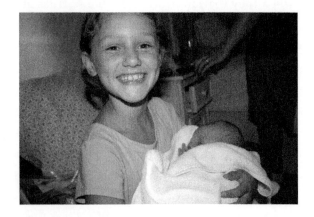

Approaching birth with this perspective can be especially intimidating to women. Before I had my eldest daughter, Kelsey, at a birth, I thought I had to have it all together for her to witness the event. I was so afraid of turning her off to birth entirely. I didn't want to scare her, but at the same time, I felt God whispering to me to be more intentional with her with regard to this birth—to leave a legacy within her by sharing this intimate time in my life with her. A legacy is created by what you do, by what you live, not just what you say. Every one leaves a legacy, either intentionally or unintentionally. I wanted to leave an intentional legacy that included her witnessing with her own eyes Mommy worshipping Jesus and surrendering all in birth. I wanted her to see what I did when I had her. I wanted to give her the gift of a vision of what birth can be when you surrender it to God. I wasn't sure how many more babies God was going to bless us with, so I felt compelled to invite her even though she was just seven years old. I wanted her to see her father and me working as a team to bring this baby into the world. I wanted her to see how God can be your strength when you are weak. I wanted to share it with her, but wondered, was she ready?

Four Tips to Decide if You Should Have Your Children at Your Birth

1) Pray about it. Ask God what He would want for your child, your birth, and your family. This decision may not be the same for every family or be wise for every child, so pray.

2) Make this decision with your husband. Is your marriage ready to have your children there? Are you going to be a good example of a team? Talking the decision over with your husband is wise; you need his support in handling the children while you are in labor if they need things (unless you choose to have other family there to help).

3) Determine whether your child is ready to be there. Is he/she personally mature enough?

4) Ask your child if she/he would like to be there and give him/her the freedom to decide.

Choosing to have your child at your birth is a deeply personal decision and one that may not be right for every family, or every child, or for every birth. As a body of Christ, this is another area where we have the opportunity to exercise respect for one another's preferences and experiences in birth.

This decision can be largely dependent on each individual's personal journey. For some women who are trained in midwifery and their children are familiar with birth as a natural occurrence in life, it may come more naturally to have their children present. For other women who have never been at another birth other than their own, the thought of having their children there might potentially stress the mother out. The father likewise may have his own thoughts and preferences with regard to what his sons and daughters see of their mother's labor and delivery. The children add an element of maturity that needs to be considered.

There are so many factors that can play into deciding whether to have a child at a birth. While this decision can cause stress in itself, ultimately, God is the one to whom you answer. If you seek Him and His guidance, He will give it to you.

If your desire is simply to serve Him in all you do in life and you have the same passion in dedicating your birth to Him, prayerfully go before His throne and seek His guidance in what He would have for this birth. Believe God has already gone before you, and He holds you and your baby in his hands.

God may be challenging you to be openly submissive in allowing Him to use this time to bring a deeper level of intimacy to a sibling relationship, a parent/child relationship, etc. As parents, we need to have a respect for the individual personal journeys each of our children are on spiritually and emotionally, but we also need to lead them. We need to seek God, humbly offering our lives to Him, submitting our wills and asking Him if He wants us to have our child at the birth or not. This decision should not be a matter of opinion. It should be based on what the Lord is clearly telling you for this birth specifically. This discernment requires being in the Word of God enough to be able to tune out all of the other words around us that so quickly entangle us from believing the truth. We need to be saturated in the Word of God and pray for guidance as we raise our children and choose which experiences to invite them into.

Every child is different and on his/her own journey toward maturity emotionally, mentally, and spiritually. We need to have a respect for that journey and not force children to be at a birth if they don't want to, or if they aren't ready. This takes being introspective about your children's lives, knowing them, their deepest fears, and so on. Listen to what God is telling you; don't decide out of fear or based on what other family members, friends, or doctors may say. Recognize that if we as parents are doing our best to teach our children openly and honestly and have a healthy relationship with them, then they would most likely want to be there. Children have a host of different thoughts and emotions about anticipating their mother giving birth. Some may have real fears that need to be talked about and going to the birth and seeing that both mommy and the baby are ok may be the exact antidote that is needed to help cure that child's fears. Fear usually comes from believing unsolicited lies or a lack of true knowledge and understanding. Often, it merely takes learning the truth about a situation to overcome a fear. The truth truly does set us free. But we need to know our children deeply—who they are. Are they anxious children in general, worrywarts? If so, then take time to help them build strength in trusting God. Devote the time necessary to lead them to the cross and grow in that area. Don't push but instead gently guide them. Only you can know your children well enough that when you go to God with their particular situations His answers give you peace either way. Discuss your thoughts about your child with your husband and ask for his insight so that you decide together.

Take a hard look at your marriage. Would having your children at your birth put an added stress on your marriage during this particular experience? Is your husband supportive and in agreement with you about the decision to have your child present or not? Are your children going to see a strong marriage working together in birth, or would having your children there make it harder and more stressful on your marriage and you while giving birth? You need to be honest with each other and prepare for this as a team. Sometimes God has a special plan for a unique experience for just husband and wife, a private time to heal and/or strengthen them.

Lastly, with regard to deciding if we should include our children in our births, we need to really take a good look at how we view birth. Why wouldn't we want them there? What lies do we believe that would keep us from being fully vulnerable in this way? What sacrifices are we afraid of making in order to have our children present? Do we truly view birth as a natural experience in life that our bodies were designed to do, or do we have fear and disbelief that things might go wrong and not want our children to see that? We ought to not ever make decisions based on fear. Fear of circumstances is not from God. What do these kinds of questions reveal about our confidence in our Creator and his design of our bodies?

Are we justifying our reason for not having our children there, when in reality we are choosing out of fear?

Birth is one of those experiences in life where God has given us the opportunity to surrender control to Him. Our culture is all about taking control of our lives to create your own destiny. We need to be careful as Christians not to accept that belief. The call for all Christians is to lay down our crosses and pick up the Lord's. We are to hate selfishness and sin, though we all struggle with it in one way or another. Raising children in today's culture is hard. The culture teaches to glorify thyself and whatever you put your mind to, you can do. We need to be in battle with these false teachings of self-doctrine (ordination). These lies seem subtle at first, but they are the seeds planted in our youth that grow into the fruit of idleness and self-glorifying proclamations. Christian parents, we need to embrace every opportunity God gives us in our ordinary lives to acknowledge Him, acknowledge His existence, and acknowledge His omniscience, His omnipotence, and His creation.

We should approach this as we would baptism, explaining it to our children and studying the Scriptures in detail to prepare them. When we have the opportunity to go to a baptism, we definitely include our children so they can witness what it looks like to be baptized and have a deeper understanding. Likewise, you can prepare your child and study the Scriptures, other books, and pray together for a deeper understanding of how God designed our bodies to have babies and how amazing He is in joining with us as we labor and as we deliver. We then can invite our children to watch us labor and deliver, with the help of God. Every birth is a spiritual experience because every baby is created and brought forth by God. We can share this amazing spiritual experience with our children. Aren't we teaching them while we sit, walk, stand, labor, sing and cry out to God, pray for strength, and praise Him? What about in that intimate time in birth when you are deeply focused, quiet, connecting with God intimately, just you two, inward . . . that quiet strength where you are battling to give control, and relinquishing control voluntarily? Do you allow your child to see you surrender all to God?

What age is appropriate?

Recognize this is not something limited by age. God never limited the younger children from coming to Him. He valued their faith deeply and told us to strive to have faith like theirs. Sometimes the encouragement that can come from the mouth of a sweet child can have the significance and wisdom of years. We need to be willing to learn from their child-like faith and trust Him like they do. Children can be refreshing to have at a birth. The innocence of their perspective is much less clouded and corrupted than ours with regard to seeing the beauty in the natural. Often their words can be such a gift when it is most needed.

Another thing to consider is that how we react and the decisions we make with regard to talking openly or not about pregnancy and childbirth directly influences our children's views of this experience—forever. We have the opportunity to leave a legacy where our children have a more confident view of God's incredible design of our bodies. And even better is the legacy of faith that can be caught by our children as they witness us living out our faith in such an intimate event in life.

I have interviewed countless women who have had their youngsters at their birth along with their midwives' babies. Birth can also be celebrated with a community of people. A dear friend shared one of her birth stories as a community celebration. She labored and gave birth outside in their hot tub in the back yard, as her two young children ran around playing with her midwife. She shared how her husband, her mother, her mother-in-law, her new sister-in-law, a dear friend, midwives, and a doula were all gathered around her together. It became a special event, bonding them all together in such an intimate way.

Our Legacy Birth Story

As we drove to the water birth center, as prepared as one can be, I still had one more decision to make. Would we have our eldest daughter Kelsey at our birth or not? She was a very mature seven year old and almost the eldest of five kids, but I wasn't 100% confident it was the right decision. Though I had given birth four times naturally, I feared I might scare her from ever having children. Though my husband assured me that I am always very considerate of others around me (labor partners) and how they are feeling while I am in labor myself, I was concerned for how a child her age might perceive it.

Months prior to my birth, I would take all my kiddos with me to my check up appointments. The midwives were so fantastic with them all. They would bring in the life-size baby figurines for them to hold and put baby powder on and diaper. They would let every child take a turn listening to the heartbeat. The midwives were always very good about making sure the kids had all their questions answered. We felt at home there. The rooms were set up like luxurious getaways—suites with a huge Jacuzzi tub, queen sized bed, and personal shower/bath. It was like a home away from home.

I was excited to give birth, but not sure if Kelsey was ready. I had spent the past seven months teaching the kids from all kinds of books on childbirth. I read them books about the development of the baby in my womb. I read them books about creation and how God made the baby in my tummy. I read them Scripture and cute little stories about adding another member to the family. When the other kids were napping, I would spend extra time and care to make sure all of her questions were answered and to read a special big girl book with her.

When the day arrived, I was still unsure of my own ability to do well having Kelsey at the birth. I was concerned I might be distracted by wanting to make sure she was okay, so after praying about it, my husband and I decided to have my sister spend the day with her nearby so she could bring her if I thought it would be appropriate.

So they came and she was such a delight to have there. I remember her knitting the baby a colorful scarf and slowly, quietly coming up to the side of the tub in between my contractions to show me the progress she had made knitting. For some reason, aside from being so proud of her, I felt a connection of relating the progress I was making in my contractions to her progress in the scarf. I found myself asking her to see how far she was on her project. It was like my progress report. Though I wasn't at home, I brought my faith and my God with me. I brought my worship music, Bounce sheets for inside my pillow (as I mentioned previously, the smell helps me calm down), and my Bible all marked up with verses I had prepared for this. I had been meditating on God's Word, singing the songs over and over at home. My husband was there to comfort me and be my strength when I needed him.

After about an hour and a half of laboring in the tub, I felt like something was different. That's how I described it, not WRONG, but DIFFERENT. My midwife tried to check. With almost certainty she said, "I think he's sunny-side up" (posterior). No wonder I had massive back pain and an intense desire to stay on all fours in the tub. Quickly my midwife ran out to the other room and came back in with a fake pelvis and a baby doll. She held the pelvis up and turned the baby's head so it would look posterior. She began to teach Kelsey what was going on so she wouldn't be scared. She gently pushed on the pelvis, inward and down dropped the baby's head. She said, "This is what we are going to do to help your mommy, is that ok with you?" Of course, the demonstration made perfect sense to her so she agreed. Immediately the midwives and Isaac took turns pushing with their knees on my pelvis. Every time they would let go to rotate and give one another a break, the pain became almost unbearable. God was so good to me. I am so thankful I had a midwife who knew just what to do in a situation like this. After a good while (about two hours) of intense labor and pushing on my pelvis while I was still on all fours in the tub, I got the urge to push. Pushing was lengthy for me, about forty-five minutes or so.

All throughout my labor, as I went from contraction to contraction, the Lord was allowing the most appropriate songs to be played on my CD player. In the moments when I could have lost my focus on Him, there was either a worship song keeping the atmosphere of the room focused on Jesus, or my husband's voice reading me specific Scriptures.

One of my fondest memories of my birth with Luke was when I was in an intense contraction, giving the midwives and Isaac a break from squeezing my pelvis together and I was floating face up in the tub, hands raised, singing worship to my Lord and Deliverer. I sang songs with all of my being through my contractions with Isaac, Kelsey, and my mother joining me in singing these songs by Selah: "Be Thou Near To Me" and "Sweet Jesus".

My contractions grew stronger and more intense. I was yearning for God. I needed Him; singing out to Him was so helpful. In the midst of an intense contraction, a song would begin and I would worship intensely. I was laboring in the waters and I felt I was in a storm. There was also a raging storm going on within me. As we sang this song, half-crying, half-singing, all those in the room listening and singing along with me, realized how the lyrics described exactly what I was experiencing. For a moment there were chuckles and laughter. God is so good. I felt His presence more than ever. He spoke to me in that moment. Those words in that song were Him speaking to me, telling me He was there with me and carrying me. I experienced a confidence, not in myself, but in the truth that He was there and He was in control.

As I would worship from one song to the next . . . God gave me the comfort, strength and will to persevere. The Lord ministered to me, connecting to me in mind, body and soul as I worshiped him. Imagine laboring in water to lyrics like these:

Just then God calmed the raging storm in me, for a moment. I was able to withdraw into myself quietly for a moment meditating on the next song, which led me to express these words through worship, "You are my hiding place, You always fill my heart with songs of deliverance, Whenever I am afraid I will trust in You," (*You Are My Hiding Place*, Selah).

"Part the Waters I Need Thee Every Hour"
By Selah

"When I cry for help, oh, hear me Lord and hold out Your hand...
Still the raging storm in me...

I need Thee every hour, in joy or pain..."

Just then progress was made, my submission to God had become complete; Luke began crowning. "Oh the Deep, Deep Love of Jesus" by Selah played, leading me to focus on the Lord, even in the pain.

Immediately following Luke's birth I held him in my arms, nursed him and rested for a few brief moments to another beautiful song by Sovereign Grace called *In the Valley* by Bob Kauflin.[*]

As I cuddled our new gift, I was in awe of our little man. And though he was covered in what most kids would have called ooey-gooey, Kelsey didn't hesitate to kiss him immediately. Standing next to the tub with enchantment on her face one of the midwives asked her, "Now how many children do you want to have?" Her reply made me so proud and I wanted to cry. With a thoughtful grin she said, "Oh, I still want as many as the Lord will give me." I hadn't scared her. If anything, I had empowered her at seven years of age.

After enjoying and bonding with Luke, I handed him to his daddy and sister as I got out of the tub. I birthed my huge healthy placenta and had a beautifully intact perineum (even after 9 lbs 9.5 oz of posterior love). I attribute that blessing to the water birth and God's mercy. Kelsey enjoyed wiping off and holding her brother before anyone else and then quickly and excitedly jumped in to help the midwives examine my placenta and then store it for later. Kelsey then volunteered to help the postpartum nurses and midwives make me a smoothie and cook me a homemade meal. She had so much fun! I was so proud of her and in awe of the bond she now had with her baby brother.

The next morning, one of my midwives came in and told me that she had never experienced such a spiritual birth and was honored to have been a part of that act of worship. Later that day our main midwife Jessica came in and showed me pictures of other posterior babies. To my surprise all the babies' heads looked oddly disfigured (which is temporary). I was shocked. Why wasn't Luke's head like this? I believe that what I endured including the pushing on my pelvis from both sides of my hips, the intense pulling, and the strong cramping while I pushed Luke out all helped to make enough room for his head. But being able to endure the pain was purely because the Lord gave me His strength as I focused on Him.

---

[*] To hear these songs and others visit redeemingchildbirth.com and go to the "Ultra Sound of Worship" tab and click play on the playlist.

Luke was born with the roundest, cute little noggin. How thankful I am that my midwives knew what to do, not only in helping me with natural pain management, but also in protecting my baby's head from too much pressure.

Most of all, I want to praise my Lord and thank Him for His grace and ability to protect us from destruction, comfort us in pain, and embrace us in trials and suffering. You see, as I surrendered my will to Him obediently in labor and delivery, God lifted me up. He chose to bless me, bless my baby, and bless my family. The memories experienced there that night and the camaraderie between the women in the family, with my mother, my sister, my daughter, my husband, and my midwives will not perish. They will be the testimonies of legacy within our family. These moments will be the experiences in life that bind us together with cords of love that cannot easily be broken.

Prayer of Thanksgiving

It's all yours, God. I surrender it all to You in praise. I am in awe of Your goodness to me. You have been faithful God to keep Your sweet promises to strengthen, empower, and teach me deep within my soul. I praise You for giving me confidence in You and Your mercies and for making me vulnerable enough to invite my daughter to participate in this amazing experience with me. I trusted in Your promises, and You did not fail me. You blessed me and blessed my family. The result of having my daughter there cannot be replaced by anything else. Our bond is greater and stronger because of You, Lord. She saw her mother in pain, but praying and praising You. And she witnessed You bring forth man from me.

Be Intentional about the Legacy You Are Leaving in Your Children

It is His design, His idea. Teach by example and model trust, faith, and confidence in the Lord. Show your children what a birth dedicated to God looks like. Engage them. Plan roles they can have in the birth. How can they participate? How can they experience this with you? Put them in charge of the music; make them the DJs. Teach them ahead of time how to change the song, so if one comes on too loudly and you need something more relaxing or quiet, they can find it for you. This is something you can train a six year old to do if you practice at home before the baby is ready to be born.

If you engage your children by letting them sing with you, pray, help by getting you a drink, watch the clock, or any other way, they will remember and learn more. The experience will mean more to them.

I have interviewed many women who have been at their mothers' births and the ones who have been involved and felt needed were the ones who themselves had a stronger memory of the event. Many who have witnessed their mothers' births also have a conviction about natural birth and view it as a normal life experience. They have a deep belief God had designed them to do this. The women who just sat back and watched, though they remembered the births, didn't share that same intimate connection with their mothers. I believe leaving an intentional legacy of faith and conviction in our children happens when we allow them to experience life with us and value them by giving them opportunities to be a team with us, to be family, working together in life.

Leaving a legacy goes beyond what legacy you leave with regard to childbirth. Everything we teach our children and do with our children (or don't do) leaves a legacy. God so desperately wants us to engage our children in every area of our lives and to impress upon them the stories, the testimonies of His goodness, His character, and His works in our lives. He wants us to invite our children to walk through life with us and purposefully allow them to see us as real people, sinful people who need a Savior. Training our children in the way they should go includes training them in how to deal with pain and how we are to respond to life transitions. The truth is, we are all weak people who need a Comforter and Protector guarding and guiding us with His supernatural strength. Our children need to see us humble and on our knees before His throne, in awe of what He has done in our lives. Our children need to see us allow God to test us and use us in order to refine us and mold us.

Our God is a loving, caring Father who wants what is best for us. He allows us to suffer, knowing that in the suffering we can experience some of our most intimate times with the Him. He wants to be intimate with you. He wants to be intimate with your children. He wants us to praise Him in the hard times and not focus on the negative so that He may strengthen us and redeem our circumstances and experiences for His glory. God has provided us the opportunity in childbearing to engage our children by mentoring them in how to surrender a life transition under the headship of Christ. Fortunately, this life transition is usually joy-filled with the added blessing of a baby.

When you have hardships, try to find God and let Him be glorified in helping you through them. And all along the way, let your children watch and walk beside you so they can learn what it means to lean on the Lord. So when they go through their own struggles and suffering in life—and they will—they will be better prepared, or at least have had a good example to learn from. Be intentional with the legacy you are leaving in all areas of life. Lean on His Word and teach your children the wisdom only found in Him. As they see you earnestly seeking Him and faithfully following Him, they will be attracted to Him as well.

Embrace the opportunity God has offered you to teach with regard to birth, life, and death. They are not to be feared, but embraced and taught.

For a free download on *Teaching Your Children about Pregnancy, Childbirth and Beyond* and a book recommendations list for teaching resources go to http://redeemingchildbirth.com/

A Heart-felt Prayer

Lord, thank You for Your Son Jesus, and that He died for our sins to be forgiven. Thank You for redeeming each of us who find our faith in You. I pray for all my sisters Lord, that they would embrace the adventure that you have in store for them in labor, pregnancy, birth and motherhood. Father, plant in all our hearts a vision for living every season of our lives intentionally. Give us belief and conviction to pursue your will in our lives, even if that means standing against the norm. Empower us with endurance and strength to engage the missions you call us to in this life.

Jesus, I pray specifically for my sisters who are with child; may you bring clarity to their mission. Guide them, give them joy when they feel it has left them. Give them courage when they feel afraid. Give them wisdom and deep conviction as they follow in surrender. Heal any brokenness in them Lord. Reconcile relationships. We ask you to prepare us all for the next season in our lives, that we may glorify You alone. Remind my sisters to be intentional about shining their lights with those that they come in contact with.

Give us the strength to do what you have made us to do with grace and thanksgiving, so that we may bring you glory. We love you Lord and are so excited for what you are going to do in the hearts of all our sisters who might read this. Please redeem childbirth in this culture, in our hearts and minds, and in your church. Please bless this project, may your hand be on it and you be magnified.

Amen.

Endnotes

1   Noah Webster, American Dictionary of the English Language, 1828.

2   Noah Webster, American Dictionary of the English Language, 1828.

3   Noah Webster, American Dictionary of the English Language, 1828.

4   Timothy Keller, *The King's Cross*, (New York: Penguin Group, 2011),16.

5   Debra Evans, *The Christian Woman's Guide to Childbirth*, Wheaton: Crossway Books, 1999), 29.

6   "Train" dictionary.refernce.com/browse/train, accessed 6-29-12.

7   "Recent decline in births in the United States, 2007–2009." http://cdc.gov/reproductivehealth/Infertility/index.htm#2, accessed, 7-10-12.

8   Dr. T. Berry Brazelton; *On Becoming a Family*, Delacorte Press, 1981.

9   Ina May Gaskin, *Ina May's Guide to Childbirth*, (New York: Bantam Dell, 2003), 134.

10 Randy Alcorn, *Heaven*, (Wheaton: Tyndale House, 2004), 16.

11 Ibid, 21.

12 "Embrace" http://dictionary.reference.com/browse/embrace, accessed 7-10-12.

13 An additional and interesting study on the history of childbirth is accurately laid out in Barbara Harper's book, *Gentle Birth Choices*.

14 Gills exposition of the Bible- http://bible.cc/genesis/3-16.htm

15 US National Library of Medicine/ National Institutes of Health- http://ncbi.nlm.nih.gov/pubmed/1756018, accessed 7-10-12.

16 Dr. Sarah J. Buckly, MD, http://sarahbuckley.com/pain-in-labour-your-hormones-are-your-helpers/, accessed 7-10-12.

17 Ibid, http://sarahbuckley.com/pain-in-labour-your-hormones-are-your-helpers/, accessed 7-10-12.

18 J.C. Ryle, *Holiness*, (Moscow, ID: Charles Nolan, 2001), 20.

19 J.I. Packer, *Concise Theology*, (Carol Stream, IL: Tyndale House, 1993), 170-171.

20 Ronnie Floyd, *How to Pray* (Nashville: Thomas Nelson, 1999), 55.

21 Richard Foster, *Prayer*, (New York: HarperCollins, 1992), 11.

22 Ibid, 12.

23 Floyd, 76.

24 Ibid.

25 Kathleen Chapman, *Teaching Kids Authentic Worship*, (Grand Rapids: Baker, 2003), 31.

26 Ibid, 29.

27 Ibid, 34.

28 Harper, Barbara, Phone Interview, January 12, 2012.

Printed in Great Britain
by Amazon

34358289R00203